# Music Has Power® in Senior Wellness and Healthcare

*of related interest*

**Musical Assessment of Gerontologic Needs and Treatment**
The MAGNET Survey
*Roberta S. Adler*
ISBN 978 1 83997 057 3
eISBN 978 1 83997 058 0

**Living Well with Dementia through Music**
A Resource Book for Activities Providers and Care Staff
*Edited by Catherine Richards*
*Foreword by Helen Odell-Miller*
ISBN 978 1 78592 488 0
eISBN 978 1 78450 878 4

**Music Therapy in a Multicultural Context**
A Handbook for Music Therapy Students and Professionals
*Edited by Melita Belgrave and Seung-A Kim*
ISBN 978 1 78592 798 0
eISBN 978 1 78450 807 4

# MUSIC HAS POWER®
# in SENIOR WELLNESS
# and HEALTHCARE

## Best Practices from Music Therapy

## Concetta Tomaino, DA, LCAT, MT-BC

Foreword by David J. Gentner, Ed.D

*This guidebook is a project of the **Institute for Music and Neurologic Function (IMNF).***

*The **Author** gratefully acknowledges the creative contribution of Joan Winer Brown, as project writer. Brown is a writer and music therapy advocate who has been associated with the IMNF more than 20 years.*

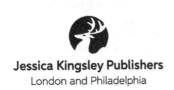

**Jessica Kingsley Publishers**
London and Philadelphia

First published in Great Britain in 2024 by Jessica Kingsley Publishers
An imprint of John Murray Press

1

A CIP catalogue record for this title is available from the
British Library and the Library of Congress

ISBN 978 1 80501 064 7
eISBN 978 1 80501 063 0

Printed and bound in the United States by Integrated Books International

Jessica Kingsley Publishers' policy is to use papers that are natural, renewable and recyclable products and made from wood grown in sustainable forests. The logging and manufacturing processes are expected to conform to the environmental regulations of the country of origin.

Jessica Kingsley Publishers
Carmelite House
50 Victoria Embankment
London EC4Y 0DZ

www.jkp.com

John Murray Press
Part of Hodder & Stoughton Limited
An Hachette UK Company

# Contents

*Foreword by David J. Gentner* . . . . . . . . . . . . . . . . 7

My Story: An Introduction to Music Therapy, and
the Institute for Music and Neurologic Function . . . . 9

**Module 1:** What is Music Therapy? . . . . . . . . . . . . . . . . . . . . 23

**Module 2:** An Introduction to Music Interventions: The
Therapeutic Drumming Circle . . . . . . . . . . . . . . . . 41

**Module 3:** Getting Started: Bringing Music Therapy Best Practices
to Your Organization . . . . . . . . . . . . . . . . . . . . . . 63

**Module 4:** Music for Mental Health and Wellness . . . . . . . . . . . 103

**Module 5:** Music for People Living with Dementia. . . . . . . . . . . 159

**Module 6:** Music for Everyday Care of People with Dementia, and
Others . . . . . . . . . . . . . . . . . . . . . . . . . . . . . . . 189

**Module 7:** Music Therapy and Movement Rehabilitation . . . . . . . 215

**Module 8:** Music Therapy and Speech Rehabilitation . . . . . . . . . . 239

Music in the Time of Covid: Challenges and
Opportunities . . . . . . . . . . . . . . . . . . . . . . . . . . 255

Technology and Virtual Programming: Expanding
Access to Music Therapy and Music Programming . . . 259

*Resources for Reference and Self-Study* . . . . . . . . . . . 271

*Acknowledgments* . . . . . . . . . . . . . . . . . . . . . . . 273

*References* . . . . . . . . . . . . . . . . . . . . . . . . . . . . 275

Accompanying materials can be found at
www.imnf.org/mhp-book-resources

# Foreword

As a lifelong senior care and housing provider, I share with you, and with colleagues in every part of our continuum, a righteous mission: to enable every older person in our care to live life to the fullest. Since 2010, I have served as President and CEO of Wartburg, a senior healthcare and housing community located on 34 beautiful acres in Westchester county, New York. We are known, in part, for our leadership in the field of creative aging. Our extensive Creative Aging and Lifelong Learning initiative offers opportunities for self-expression, growth, and joy to older people, many of whom are coping with cognitive or physical challenges.

In 2018, Wartburg became home to the Institute for Music and Neurologic Function (IMNF), an internationally recognized authority on music therapy, research, and training. The IMNF has more than 25 years of clinical experience in using music therapy to improve the level of function and quality of life for people with Alzheimer's disease and other forms of dementia, Parkinson's disease, and the disabilities caused by stroke or traumatic brain injury.

At the same time, we recognize that it is important to extend the benefits of music programming to the well seniors in our independent living apartments, and those living in assisted living, many of whom have cognitive impairments. Our mission, after all, is to enable *every* person in our care to live life to the fullest, to live their "best life" at Wartburg. Research shows us that music therapy is highly effective in addressing the challenges of aging. For example, engagement in music is a powerful way of helping older people cope with depression in response to inevitable losses; with anxiety about change, and the future; with lack of cognitive stimulation; and with social withdrawal.

At Wartburg, we are pioneers, perhaps the first regional senior healthcare and housing provider to integrate music therapy techniques into care and rehabilitation across our community, so that the therapeutic powers of music will become available to all who can benefit.

What is our larger goal? To bring the best practices in music therapy—and the healing power of music—beyond Wartburg's campus, to you, and to build a regional research base with international collaborations.

*David J. Gentner, Ed.D*

# My Story: An Introduction to Music Therapy, and the Institute for Music and Neurologic Function

## CONCETTA ("CONNIE") TOMAINO

"Born and raised in New York City, the daughter of a green-grocer and what was then called a 'stay at home' mom..." That's how my story begins. Music was there from the beginning, for as long as I can remember. As a small child, I was always playing with sounds and making up songs. Later, I would drag the record player outdoors and my friends and I would stage "lip sync" versions of musicals in my garage—our driveway was on a hill which it made it perfect for theatrical seating (though none of us had ever been to a real theater). By second grade, I was singing in the church choir and beginning to notice musical instruments. One of my neighbors played the accordion, and I spent many hours in his yard, sitting at his knees and listening to him play. It was magical.

Of course, I desperately wanted to take music lessons. My parents were at first unable to afford this, but then, when I was ten years old, it became possible. At first it was thought that I would take piano or guitar lessons, as so many other children did. But I was drawn to the accordion. It became my instrument. I took lessons and practiced rigorously for six years. Later the trumpet would become my instrument of choice for study and performance. But to this day it is the accordion that is my main choice for music therapy.

*I am sharing this brief bio with you as an introduction to music therapy. But in a larger sense I want to persuade you that it is your life that is the best introduction to music therapy and what it can do. If at this moment I were to approach you as a music therapist, perhaps with my accordion, I would be able to call on the music that you know and remember, the music that is part of your identity, the music that is indestructibly encoded in your brain. This is the music that you will be able to respond to, physically and emotionally, as long as you live.*

*Your music, like mine, includes the music of childhood. In fact, the familiar songs of our childhood, teenage, and young adult years tend to bring forth the strongest responses and memories in us. So as you read my story, I hope you will take a moment to listen to the music of your beginnings as well. At family gatherings. On YouTube. Or in your own mind—because the music is still there.*

## Music and medicine

I didn't set out to become a music therapist, or even a professional musician. My original goal was to become a medical doctor. I was a real science geek, and planned to focus on science during my high school and college years. Unknowingly, I was on a path to both music and medicine, in ways that I could not then imagine.

In high school, I joined the band, choosing the trumpet. As a child, I had heard live performances by Louis Armstrong and Count Basie at Free-domland, a short-lived theme park in the Bronx. I knew that if I were to play another instrument it would be the trumpet. Soon I had opportunities to play in ensembles—including pep bands playing Dixieland and Tijuana Brass tunes; brass quartets for church service, marching bands, and wind ensembles. In my senior year of high school, I began playing with the Bronx House Symphony Orchestra, a community orchestra of semi-professional musicians, and my first real exposure to the classical repertoire.

When I entered college (the first woman in my family to do so), it was as a biology major/pre-med. I chose the State University of New York (SUNY) at Stony Brook because then, as now, it had a rich music culture, in which I hoped to participate. But the college music department was similar to a conservatory, and because I did not have a strong background in contemporary classical music—but played everything more or less intuitively—some opportunities were closed to me, at least at first. Eventually, I was guided to a talented trumpet teacher who prepared me to go forward, in my sophomore year, as a double major, biology-pre-med and music.

Which would it be? Medicine or music? It was a serious internal conflict for me, made more difficult by the situational challenges of the pre-med curriculum, and the growing awareness that I needed to immerse myself in music. By my third year, I had decided to switch my major to trumpet performance.

## The "new field" of music therapy

It was about this time that I came across an article, in a teen magazine(!), about "the new field of music therapy." There was, it seemed, a profession that would allow me to combine my two passions—music and healthcare. I learned that New York University (NYU) had just started a music therapy program, and this encouraged me to interview and audition for the Master's Program in Music Therapy. To prepare, I began taking psychology courses, and got permission to do an independent study in child development and music. A month after graduating from Stony Brook, I began studies at NYU.

As a music therapist, my instruments would be mainly the accordion and piano. I was told upfront that there were no trumpet-playing music therapists—and there are reasons for this. You cannot sing (or talk) while playing the trumpet, and you cannot easily hold another with your eyes. The accordion allows closer interactions, and seems to breathe along with you and the client. It has remained my instrument of choice as a therapist. Thankfully, I continued to have many opportunities to play the trumpet while at NYU, in wind ensembles, jazz groups, and rehearsal bands throughout the city.

At NYU, I had the privilege of working with Professor Barbara Hesser, as her first graduate assistant. At that time, Hesser's office also served as headquarters for the American Association for Music Therapy (AAMT), one of two national professional organizations for music therapists and students. (The two organizations merged in 1998 to form the American Music Therapy Association (AMTA).) I was the first student representative on the AAMT Board of Directors, with the founders of that organization, and I helped organize the AAMT annual conferences, which were held at NYU. The association was growing; I was learning not only music therapy, but also the business skills that would serve me well through my career.

## Music therapy—and first discoveries

During my second year at NYU (I completed the Master's in three years), I had a paid internship in a skilled nursing facility in East New York (in Brooklyn). It was here that I first witnessed the ability of music to reach people with late-stage Alzheimer's disease. These individuals were said to have "no minds left." And yet a familiar song calmed their agitation, and many responded by singing the words of the song. This was a startling discovery that raised profound questions. I wondered how someone with "no brain function," no cognitive function, could process the sound as a melody and remember the words. I wanted to know what it was about music that was so meaningful, so well preserved, that those who seemed unreachable could be reached through music. At the skilled nursing facility, I also worked with stroke survivors in the rehabilitation of motor and communication skills. Here, too, music seemed to have important therapeutic effects. (My Master's thesis explored stroke rehabilitation with music therapy, in greater depth.) *All of this was new, to me, to everyone.* It was 1978, and little was known about the recovery of function after brain injury or stroke. The research at that time offered no explanation for why music had these effects on neurological function.

## Oliver Sacks: Awakenings

In summer 1978, my father died; I was living at home and needed a full-time job to help the family meet expenses. Full-time jobs for music therapists were rare in those days, but in 1979 I answered an advert in the local paper and was hired by a skilled nursing home in the Bronx, on the street where my father had worked for his whole life.

Within my first weeks on the job, I received an inter-office envelope, addressed "to the music therapist." Enclosed was a torn piece of loose-leaf paper with these words, scribbled:

> "Every disease is a musical problem. Every cure a musical solution" (Novalis).
> Welcome, Ollie

I soon learned that Ollie was Oliver Sacks, MD, the consulting neurologist, who was said to be eccentric and a little asocial, but very caring with patients. He wrote endless medical notes: every patient was a person he was truly concerned about, and he seemed to want to capture the essence of who they were and how to best help them. It seemed too good to be true—that there was a medical doctor who recognized the importance of music. I looked for an opportunity to meet him.

I wanted to ask: if every disease is a musical problem, what about Alzheimer's and dementia? What about stroke...what about..."every disease?"

Not long after I received the note, I saw one of the residents with late-stage dementia outside Dr. Sacks's office. So I waited, and when Dr. Sacks arrived, I introduced myself and told him I had been working with his patient. He asked me to bring her into his office. He gently took her to a comfortable space and softly sang, "Daisy, Daisy, give me your answer do." And he got her to smile and nod, holding her hand and singing to her, which is something I couldn't imagine any other neurologist doing. But I knew she could go further, and I offered this resident music that had meaning to her, a gospel song from her childhood. And we saw, Dr. Sacks and I, that this music therapy intervention not only helped our patient to sing—a clinical miracle in itself—but also brought her into the moment, lucidly speaking about herself, remembering how she felt, and where she was when she heard this song. Dr.

Sacks—Oliver—was fascinated, both as a neurologist, and on behalf of his patients. And thus began our work together.

## Questions—and discoveries

I looked for more opportunities to meet with Oliver, to ask him questions and share patient stories. And he made it a point to refer patients to me. He shared his immense learning, in neurology and evolutionary science, and the literature of medical science; I shared my experience as a music therapist, seeking to understand and apply the new and powerful ideas of music therapy and neuroscience to the lives of the patients before us.

I was moved, more than once, by the way Oliver sometimes deferred to me, in clinical matters, despite his much greater knowledge in medicine and neurology. It seemed that he realized that in some cases—so many cases—the disease was a musical problem in the deepest sense, encompassing the brain functions associated with the processing of rhythm and movement, and harmony and melody. And that the solution, the therapy that worked, might be music therapy.

Oliver lived on City Island, a community on a small island in Long Island Sound that was part of my bicycle ride back to my home in the Bronx. We sometimes met at his house, as part of his project to introduce me, the new music therapist, to the world of neurology. For each question I had, Oliver pulled a book from his collection of first editions (Henry Head, John Hughlings Jackson, Charles Darwin...) and introduced me to the founding fathers of neurology and evolutionary science. He gave me copies of A.R. Luria's book *The Man with a Shattered World* (Luria, 1971/1987) as an introduction to how a damaged mind must reconstruct the world to be engaged with it. And much more: he gave me, and the world too, his own accounts of the patients he treated for "damaged minds" or neurological disorders. What he wanted from me—and what I wanted to give—were clinical applications of music therapy to real patients, in real healthcare settings. And he understood, we both did, that this would be based in neuroscience as a scientific and humanistic discipline.

On the days that Dr. Sacks came to the nursing home ("Beth Abraham") we would discuss music and our patients on lunchtime walks at the Botanical Gardens, nearby. He shared the journals of his awakening patients—people I was now working with. All of this fueled my desire to learn more about music and the brain.

## Progress

Increasingly, Oliver and I had opportunities to discuss various patients when he was updating their assessment and progress. He would often ask: How was the patient in music? Can she initiate a beat? Repeat a melody? Sing words? I set out to observe every nuance of a patient's response to music. Where did it initiate? Was it mimicry or interactive? I was beginning to see how various neurologic impairments could alter a person's perception of music as well as influence their capacity for non-music-based responses. As Oliver and I shared information and insights on a weekly basis, we began to realize that *there was something about music—the auditory system and its connections—that could restore function to those with severe neurologic impairments.*

Other clinicians were beginning to observe these effects. In the very first issue of the journal *Music Therapy*, in 1981, an article by music therapist Alice Rogers and speech language pathologist Paul Fleming, working out of a Veterans Affairs hospital in Cincinnati, described a music intervention that was effective in helping stroke patients recover speech. Some stroke patients with non-fluent aphasia, who were unable to speak, could sing or hum familiar songs—and that ability to sing, preserved in the injured brain, provided a path to speech rehabilitation. This work, which was grounded in neuroscience, was very similar to what we were doing—and the results were encouraging and validating.

But the work was new, and the field of music therapy was little known in the medical and scientific community. Our work, too, remained largely unknown, except among a few clinicians at the very few healthcare institutions that had a music therapist on staff. We needed a better plan.

In 1984, Oliver and I met with several scientists to discuss the feasibility of studying music and the brain. We were told that music was too complex to study neurologically; that the recovery of function that we were seeing in our patients was transient; that the brain doesn't recover lost functions. As clinicians on the frontlines, we knew that this was not true.

At our nursing home in the Bronx we saw patients with late-stage dementia who were unable to communicate until music unlocked their memories and their words. We saw stroke patients with non-fluent aphasia for whom the ability to sing, preserved in the injured brain, provided a path to speech rehabilitation. I began taking courses in neuroscience at Columbia, and when I returned to NYU for a doctorate I wanted to do my dissertation on music and memory. But the neuroscience was not there yet, and I was advised to study further my own clinical work with people with dementia. My dissertation investigated preserved memories elicited by autobiographical music.

Again, the message was clear; in time science would have much to tell us about music and the brain. For now, what we needed was clinical experience and clinical research.

## Recognition—and a vision for the future

In the late 1980s, I had become president of AAMT, afterwards serving on various task forces that were defining the scope of music therapy. Additionally, I had begun networking with the music industry as potential partners in music therapy. This involved meeting with representatives from Yamaha, Remo, and Roland, for example, to find ways of incorporating new music technologies into music therapy.

During this time, Oliver had become a publishing phenomenon—a best-selling author who captured the imagination of a wide audience. *The Man Who Mistook his Wife for a Hat*, Oliver's breakthrough book, was published in 1985; *Awakenings*, which told the stories of patients at Beth Abraham, was an award-winning film in 1990. Both of us were being interviewed for radio and TV programs. This drew the attention of the president of our facility. Why were media from around the world coming to meet with us? Why, all at once, was music in a nursing home so important? I was invited to speak to the Beth Abraham Board of Directors, to explain that music was more than an activity; that the ability to respond to music seemed to be uniquely preserved in the brain; and that we were able to use music to help restore neurological function in many of our patients.

The message was beginning to get across, at least in the wider world. In 1990, I received a call from an aide to Senator Harry Reid, who had heard an interview by Mickey Hart of the Grateful Dead in which he spoke about his grandmother's Alzheimer's disease. The Older Americans Act was up for revision, a hearing was scheduled—and "everyone on Capitol Hill was a deadhead"—"so how do we get Mickey to Washington?" The hearing before the Special Committee on Aging, which took place on August 1, 1991, focused entirely on music and aging. Mickey spoke about the importance of rhythm and drumming for those with dementia. Oliver gave clinical examples and a videotape presentation that made music therapy come alive to the Committee, through the experiences of our patients. The hearing was a huge success, leading to research grants in music therapy.

# "The power of music is fundamental . . ."

*From the testimony of Dr. Oliver Sacks, Neurologist, Senate*
*Special Committee on Aging, August 1, 1991*

Finally, and most importantly: those patients—whose numbers now, tragically, run into the millions—those patients with a dementia due to the diffuse cortical damage of Alzheimer's disease, patients who may be in a pitiful state of agitation and confusion because their memories and powers to organize are failing, because they *cannot* hold themselves and their worlds together. The power of music is fundamental, with such patients...it acts as a sort of Proustian mnemonic, eliciting emotions and associations which have been long forgotten, giving the patient access, once again to moods and memories and worlds which, seemingly, they have completely lost. One sees that it is not an actual loss of memories here, but a loss of *access* to these—and music, above all, can provide access once again, can constitute a key for opening the door to the past, a door not only to specific memories, but to the entire thought structure and personality of the past.

Thus, with music—and here, above all, it must be the "right" music, the music which holds significance, has meaning for the individual—the patient with dementia can be *restored to himself*; can recall, re-access, not only his powers of speech, his perceptual and thinking skills, but his entire emotional and intellectual configuration, his life history, his identity—for a while. It is incredibly poignant to see such recalls, such restorations of the otherwise lost persona.

## The Institute for Music and Neurologic Function (IMNF)

With recognition and more funding coming to music therapy, there were new opportunities to conduct clinical research and disseminate findings through the healthcare system.

At this time, our music therapy program had a champion in Arnold Goldstein, a seasoned hospital administrator as well as a talented songwriter. Goldstein undertook to help me and Oliver achieve new funding for research and conference events. In 1993, we organized a conference entitled "Clinical Applications of Music in Neurologic Rehabilitation," which was attended by more than 125 music therapists. In addition to disseminating research, the conference introduced new technologies in rehabilitation, including "soundbeam" and computer-based interfaces. The event so impressed Beth Abraham's president that he announced that we would be establishing an institute to advance music therapy research and training, through the study of music and the brain.

The same year, 1993, Oliver and I were awarded a substantial grant by the New York State Department of Health (NYSDOH) to study music and memory in people with Alzheimer's disease, in collaboration with a neurologist at the Albert Einstein College of Medicine. I was promoted to the Department of Medicine, and was able to hire a full-time music therapist. Other grants and collaborations followed. With the realization that we could attract significant funding, we were able to formalize the legal incorporation of the Institute for Music and Neurologic Function, in 1995, with Arnold as its first executive director. The IMNF was a separate 501(c) (3) organization, with its own Board of Directors.

The new Institute for Music and Neurologic Function was unique in being located within a long-term healthcare system. This meant that we were able to develop music therapy programs and conduct research on clinical outcomes in music therapy, at the same time. Our impact extended well beyond our own institution, as those of us associated with the IMNF—myself, Oliver, and later many others—participated in collaborations and presented our research at numerous medical and geriatric conferences across the nation. We also gave workshops on therapeutic uses of music in dementia care, and in time began a training program for music therapy students. From the beginning, the Institute also maintained a network of friends and supporters in the music industry; we were early adapters of music-based technology in rehabilitation.

## "Dialogues across disciplines"

An important breakthrough for the IMNF was a grant from the US Administration on Aging to investigate best practices for dementia care and stroke rehabilitation. This grant represented not only national recognition but also support of close to half a million dollars, a large grant at that time. Funding for a symposium was included in the grant, so that the IMNF's work could be widely disseminated. The Dialogues Across Disciplines symposium, in 2002, brought together neuroscientists and music therapists in the US and beyond, to share their work. Speakers, all leaders in their various fields, included Karl Pribram, Robert Zatorre, Mark Tramo, Gottfried Schlaug, Larry Parsons, Michael Thaut, Wendy Magee, and David Ramsey. By 2005, the IMNF was truly reaching across disciplines, and expanding its connections with the neuroscience community. We were also providing in-services and training for national organizations, such as the National Alzheimer's Foundation, the MS Society, the Parkinson's Disease Foundation, and others.

In many ways, the IMNF was expanding beyond our Beth Abraham base.

And Beth Abraham was expanding, and changing too, becoming "Bethco," then "CenterLight." In 2008, the IMNF's corporate funding ended. The new entity, CenterLight, now had four nursing homes and a large managed home-care program, so there was an opportunity for the IMNF to provide contract services throughout the system. The contract with the homecare program expanded music therapy services, and allowed me to train caregivers and music therapy staff in a changing healthcare environment. This preserved the integrity of the music therapy program for another eight years until changes in the Medicaid reimbursement caused CenterLight to greatly reduce music therapy hours.

The IMNF continues to provide services to CenterLight, to this day; and we have also created an outpatient practice to serve the community. But, in 2015, it became clear that we needed a new home—a home that would allow us to help greater numbers of patients, and strengthen our focus on research collaborations.

## The IMNF at Wartburg

Finding a supportive partner for the IMNF became a two-year journey. We knew that our work provided opportunities, at the clinical level, to transform the lives of seniors in long-term care, and in our communities.

We had shown, through IMNF research, the power of music to improve the care, and the quality of life, for people with depression, dementia, stroke, and other disorders. So we asked ourselves—how can we bring what we have learned into medical practice and the healthcare system? Should we become part of a university, a medical school, a hospital? Each option offered opportunities for advancing our work. But only if we could find the right leadership. Finding an empowered administrator who really shared the IMNF's vision was a challenge. That is until I met David Gentner, President and CEO of Wartburg, a senior care community in Mount Vernon, New York.

I was introduced to David by a colleague I greatly respected, who had been recruited to head Wartburg's Adult Day program. My colleague told me that David was an empathetic leader who truly valued staff input; and he was known to have a special interest in music and the creative arts in care-giving. I learned that David had chosen for his doctoral dissertation to study the effect of music programming on seniors in assisted living; that he had observed first hand the responses of people with dementia to familiar music and other interventions; and that he wanted to apply what he was learning to the seniors in his care. This being so, I should not have been surprised to learn that he had followed my work and the IMNF for some time, but I was truly moved by this. At our first meeting, we were talking about the future, and a vision that we shared.

At Wartburg, David had created the Council on Creative Aging and Lifelong Learning as an initiative that would combine the arts and science to create an environment for healthy aging. This had evolved into an award-winning program and international model. Now David and his senior staff wanted to expand the model to include creative arts therapies. They had already established a dance therapy program and the beginnings of a music therapy program. David invited me to meet with senior staff and discuss the potential of the IMNF moving to Wartburg, to create a state-of-the-art music therapy program for the people in the Wartburg community. Everyone was enthusiastic and supportive.

More quickly than I could have imagined, everything seemed to fall into place. I witnessed David's willingness to help out when I received notice that all the IMNF's equipment had to be claimed immediately. I called David to see if he had any storage space. Despite the fact that we had not formalized the IMNF's move to Wartburg, David was willing not only to offer free storage space but also to come with his engineering staff to move the equipment for me and our envisioned program. I had never seen an administrator offer to "do the work" himself. I knew that anyone willing to help at this level would be an honest and dedicated person to work with.

Wartburg's core mission is to enable seniors to live life to the fullest, through integrated healthcare and housing which nurture body, mind, and spirit—and this resonated with me. Because of its continuum of care, Wartburg offered opportunities to include music therapy in outpatient rehabilitation, skilled nursing, memory care, and well aging. I also learned that Wartburg had close ties with local colleges offering opportunities for student training and research collaborations. These connections, and the spirit in which they were put forward, went far beyond what I had seen in any other senior-serving organization. It seemed that the IMNF had found a home that would support therapy for seniors, as well as training and research that had the potential to improve the quality of life for the growing numbers of seniors (and caregivers) who would need care in the future.

In 2017, as the IMNF moved to Wartburg, David wrote, "The goal now is to bring best practices in music therapy and therapeutic aspects of music beyond Wartburg's campus and build a strong regional research base with international collaborations, including music therapy training and increased donor support." This best practices guidebook is part of our effort to fulfill this mission.

Interestingly, Wartburg was the name of the facility in East New York where my journey in music and memory first began in 1978. I felt as if I had come full circle and the IMNF's new home base would provide renewed growth and mission.

# IMNF timeline

## Major grant-funded research and projects of the Institute for Music and Neurologic Function (IMNF)

**1993**

Beth Abraham Health Services hosts its first international music therapy conference, "Clinical Applications of Music in Neurologic Rehabilitation," and announces a plan to create an institute dedicated to exploring music and the brain.

Beth Abraham music therapists, in collaboration with the neuroscience division of the Albert Einstein College of Medicine, and with funding from Wallerstein Foundation for Geriatric Life Improvement, begin investigating music and neurophysiology, verbal memory, and recovery of function in the auditory system.

The New York State Department of Health (NYSDOH) Dementia Grant Program funds Beth Abraham's music therapy program to research the effects of music on memory in persons with dementia.

**1995**

IMNF is formally incorporated.

IMNF receives an NYSDOH grant to study "Effects of a music therapy intervention on the levels of depression, anxiety/agitation, and quality of life experienced by individuals diagnosed with early and middle stage dementias."

Haym Salomon Geriatric Foundation funds research on the effects of music therapy in people with dysarthria.

**1997**

Scheuer Family Foundation funds music therapy group programs for persons with dementia.

**1998**

Scheuer Family Foundation funds a demonstration project on the efficacy of using musical instrument digital interface (MIDI) equipment to reinforce occupational therapy goals—the genesis of the Music Has Power recording studio.

**2002**

US Administration on Aging awards the IMNF $493,000 for "Innovative Music/Neurologic Approaches to Improve Quality and Effectiveness in Stroke and Dementia Care."

IMNF holds international symposium "Dialogues Across Disciplines: Cognitive Neuroscience and Music Processing in Human Function," bringing together neuroscientists and clinicians for the first time.

**2004**

United Hospital Fund grant supports production of training video used to deliver therapeutic music programs for people with Alzheimer's and dementia.

Christopher Reeve Paralysis Foundation supports a recording studio rehabilitation program.

**2005**

New York State Department of Health (NYSDOH) funds the IMNF to develop therapeutic drumming outreach and training programs.

**2007**

In fulfillment of the NYSDOH grant, a workshop on "Rhythm and Drumming Activities for Dementia Care" provides training to NYC area healthcare professionals.

**2008**

IMNF begins New York Community Trust grant research on the impact of music therapy on depression and apathy, in conjunction with Beth Abraham's Comprehensive Care Management (CCM) programs.

**2009**

Through a Fan Fox & Leslie R. Samuels Foundation grant, the IMNF, working with its CCM sites, launches a two-year research project to examine the efficacy of music therapy for outpatient and in-home care and to assess if there are benefits for caregivers as well.

**2010**

IMNF begins development of a comprehensive music therapy evaluation scale to look at a patient's general mental state, self-evaluation, pain, motor function, speech/language function, cognition, psychosocial function, and more.

IMNF studies use of familiar songs and rhythmic speech motor entrainment for speech improvement among patients with non-fluent aphasia.

**2011**

IMNF evaluates the effect of a variety of music-based interventions to improve communication outcomes in persons with non-fluent aphasia.

**2013**

A study on the effects of music therapy on short-term memory on patients with Alzheimer's disease is carried out with a medical student at SUNY Stony Brook.

**2016**

IMNF partners with the Louis Armstrong Music and Medicine Center at Mount Sinai along with Lincoln Center to study the impact of a specialized audience program for persons with dementia and their care partners.

**2018**

The ASCAP Foundation provides funding for the IMNF's Music Therapy Clinic for Asphasia, as part of its continuing support for the IMNF.

**2020**

IMNF receives a grant from the Scott Amrhein Memorial Fund to support a guide to best practices in music therapy-informed programs for senior health and well-being.

**2022**

IMNF launches Music Has Power® for Parkinson's, a program supported by a community grant from the Parkinson's Foundation.

# MODULE 1

# What is Music Therapy?

Chances are, you already know and understand a lot about music therapy. Even if you're not familiar with the use of music in healthcare, you have likely experienced some of the therapeutic benefits of music in your own life. What's more, you may have used music therapy techniques, naturally, without even realizing it, to provide love and care to others.

## ABOUT YOU

1. What experience do you bring to music therapy?

_____

_____

Have you ever met or worked alongside a music therapist?
Yes     No     Don't know

Have you observed a music therapist engaging in music with an individual, or with a group?
Yes     No     Don't know

Have you ever seen a music therapist portrayed in a film or video? If so, please specify.

_____

If you have observed a music therapist in practice (or on film or video), describe what you observed, and what if anything did you learn from the experience?

_____

_____

## TAKEAWAY

If you have never met a music therapist, you are not alone. There are only about 10,000 music therapists in the US. If you have met a music therapist in a healthcare, school, or mental health setting, you've had an experience most Americans haven't had. The shortage of music therapists is a problem in our healthcare system. That's why music therapists are passionate about sharing their knowledge and skills with others, so as to increase access to music therapy across the healthcare system, and in other settings.

2. Music therapy brings together the words "music" and "therapy."

*What does the word "music" mean to you?*

Have you played a musical instrument, at any time in your life? If so, what do you remember about this experience?

_____

_____

What were your goals, in learning to play a musical instrument? (For example, parental praise, performances at recitals, acceptance into an ensemble or jazz group, mastery of certain techniques or compositions.)

_____

Did you sing in a school or community chorus, or a religious choir? If so, what do you remember about this experience?

_____

What were your goals as a singer or choir member? (For example, parental praise, fun with peers, performances at recitals, events, religious services; solo opportunities; mastery of certain techniques or vocal compositions.)

_____

_____

*What does the word "therapy" mean to you?*

Have you (or has someone you know) received physical therapy? If so, what were the goals of this physical therapy? (For example, regain function after an injury or after surgery, overcome pain, improve range of motion.)

_____

Have you (or has someone you know) received psychotherapy or counseling from a mental health professional? If so, what were the goals of psychotherapy or counseling? (For example, relieve anxiety, overcome depression, increase self-esteem or motivation.)

_____

_____

## TAKEAWAY

Your goals, when you were a music student—playing a musical instrument in elementary school, and maybe even into the college years—were partly music goals, relating to music learning, performance, and mastery. And no doubt you had other goals as well. *Music therapy is not about achieving music goals. It's about therapy*, improving health and well-being through music.

Music therapists are trained musicians, proficient in numerous instruments and in music composition and improvisation. Any music training you've had will likely increase your understanding of the work they do. But you don't need to have a music background in order to take ideas and techniques from music therapy and apply them in caregiving. That can happen when music therapists share their knowledge and skills with others in the healthcare team (as we will do here).

## TAKEAWAY

The goals that you have identified for physical therapy and psychotherapy are very similar to the goals of music therapy. And music therapy offers uniquely effective ways of achieving these goals. For example, music therapy, like physical therapy, helps patients regain function after a stroke or traumatic brain injury, often when other medical interventions have failed. Music therapy, like psychotherapy, addresses depression and anxiety. Music therapy also provides avenues for communication for people who are unable to express themselves in words, due to depression, serious mental illnesses, or dementia, for example.

Some people don't have a history of making music, or singing, and some have not had an experience with therapy or counseling. But nearly everyone listens to music. If you do:

How many hours a day do you listen to music? (Provide an estimate.)

_____

Where do you generally listen to music? (For example, at home, in the car, at parties, in earphones at work, running, or at exercise in the gym.)

_____

_____

What are your wellness goals in listening to music? That is, what positive effects do you expect to get out of the listening experience?

I am not aware of any goals in listening to music.

My goals are the following. (For example, a lift in spirits, or improved mood, relaxation, improved sleep quality, relief of boredom, better performance in social settings, support for exercise, entertainment.)

_____

_____

As you think about the ways you listen to music, can you remember any ways in which listening to music has sometimes contributed to a negative outcome for you? (For example, brought to mind memories you couldn't cope with, sapped your motivation for work, caused you to drink too much, drive too fast, or engage in other risky behaviors?)

_____

## TAKEAWAY

Listening to music may be therapeutic—but not always. For example, listening to music in order to achieve a relaxed state or quality sleep may be therapeutic; it may even reduce the experience of chronic pain, if that is a concern. Listening to music, passively, for its entertainment value, is less likely to be therapeutic, in the sense of helping you meet wellness goals. Music listening, to be therapeutic, ideally should be guided by a music therapist or other healthcare professional who understands your goals and healthcare needs.

## TAKEAWAY

There are very few contraindications for using music to help meet health and wellness goals. Music has power—even for people who can't easily be reached in any other way. And yet a piece of music can sometimes bring to mind negative images and memories, leading to depression. Music in a particular setting can provide the soundtrack for addiction or other self-harming behaviors, and so forth. It is important that the music a person experiences is the right music (or the right kind of music) at the right time. In our own lives, we tend to know to use music to manage our moods and behaviors. As caregivers in senior care, we rely on music therapists to help us recognize when the music offered to a person is not the right music; or when, in rare instances, music therapy is contraindicated.

Music therapists have created online resources to share their knowledge, skills, and experience. To learn more about music therapy and the Institute for Music and Neurologic Function, visit www.imnf.org/mhp-book-resources.

## Music therapy: A simple definition

Music therapy is a form of therapy in which a board-certified music therapist (MT-BC) establishes a therapeutic relationship with an individual (or a group of individuals) and uses music to improve their health and well-being.

Music therapy is the term applied when services are provided by a professional music therapist. But we should note that there are therapeutic uses of music that have been consistently shown to be effective, and can be used by other members of the healthcare team. For example, over the years, music therapists discovered that music, especially familiar songs, can help people with dementia access memories and emotions. Today, other members of the healthcare team are incorporating familiar songs into memory care—with excellent results.

A simple definition, as applied to senior care, might be:

Music therapy is a form of healthcare that is provided to older people to support their health and wellness, rehabilitation, and memory care, through engagement with music. Music therapy techniques are adapted to meet the needs of older people (and their caregivers) across a continuum of care settings, ranging from independent living to long-term care.

Here are some examples of how music therapy is applied to the challenges of aging:

- A music therapist sings familiar songs to residents in a long-term facility, engaging them to join in with rhythm instruments, as a way of connecting to one another.

- A music therapist prescribes an exercise that uses rhythmic music to help a person with Parkinson's disease regulate their gait and motor function.

- A nurse consults with the music therapist and prescribes music to help a nursing home patient manage chronic pain.

- A recreation therapist in an adult day-care program consults with a music therapist on how to use music as a "memory tool," while providing a fun activity.

- A home health aide uses music therapy techniques with a person with dementia to create moments of pleasurable interaction around daily activities, such as dressing and bathing.

- A trained musician volunteer gives a workshop for seniors who used to play musical instruments, and collaborates with them to create original pieces reflecting their ideas.

The examples above are drawn from the healthcare experiences with older people. But to understand the power of music to improve the lives of older people, you need to know how **music affects the health and well-being of people at all stages of life**—because people with dementia, like you and me, carry within them the needs and experiences that they have had over the course of a lifetime:

- In the neonatal intensive care unit (NICU), the right music can help stabilize the premature infant's heart and breathing rate. Parents are able to bond with their infants as they participate in music stimulation, by singing lullabies, for example.

- For children and adults with autism spectrum disorder and intellectual disabilities, music therapy often helps them achieve their full potential. (In fact, almost as many music therapists work in children's facilities and schools as in geriatric facilities.)

- Across adolescence and adulthood, music therapy is often an effective treatment for depression, addiction, and identity issues; for traumatic brain injuries incurred in accidents, sports accidents, or military service; and for serious psychiatric illness, such as major depression, bi-polar disorder, and post-traumatic stress disorder (PTSD).

- And at the end of life, music therapy is often included as part of the Medicare hospice care plan, in recognition of its effectiveness in relieving both psychological distress and physical pain.

**Music therapy also has many applications for people who simply want to achieve a higher level of well-being—greater creativity, more resilience in the face of life's demands, or simply a deep and reliable pleasure, accessible at will, to help them cope from day to day.**

## A closer look

The official definition of the AMTA (American Music Therapy Association) is:

Music therapy is the clinical and evidence-based use of music interventions to accomplish individualized goals within a therapeutic relationship by a credentialed professional who has completed an approved music therapy program.

Let's unpack this definition, to see how it applies to our needs as providers of senior care:

- **The word "clinical" means that music therapy is provided directly to individuals as part of medical treatment, rehabilitation, and caregiving.** Music that is provided as recreation or entertainment is not "clinical" in this sense, and is not music therapy. Nevertheless, "the more music, the better" is an attitude adopted by most music therapists. An environment that offers music in all its forms is in the best position to develop a music therapy program.

- **The words "evidence based" mean that music therapy is based on documented clinical experience and scientific research, including studies that measure the outcome of music interventions.** A music therapist decides to offer a music intervention, such as singing or listening to familiar music on an iPod, not because it is popular among residents of a senior care facility (though it often is), but because there is *evidence* that this intervention, for a particular individual or class of individuals, is likely to achieve a therapeutic goal that can be measured. For example, the intervention might reduce anxiety or pain, or improve quality of life in measurable ways.

  Researchers have developed ways to measure and objectively observe the outcomes of music interventions. They use assessment tools, such as the Alzheimer's Disease-Related Quality of Life instrument (ADRQL), the Geriatric Depression Scale (GDS), as well as structured interviews with patients and their caregivers. A well-designed research study will compare the outcomes of those who receive a music therapy intervention with an equivalent or carefully matched group of people who receive a different intervention or no intervention at all. Findings from such studies form the basis for music therapy practice. Well-documented case studies are also part of the evidence base.

- **Music therapy seeks to accomplish "individualized goals within a therapeutic relationship."** At the core of best practices in music therapy is the therapeutic relationship between an individual who is seeking help and support (the patient or client), and the music therapist. The concept of the therapeutic relationship is basic to many forms of therapy; key elements of the relationship include trust, empathy, respect, and care, among others. In music therapy, the therapist and patient engage with music *together*—listening to music together, making music together, improvising music together; and then perhaps talking about what the music means to the patient or client. This sharing and interacting with music in real time creates a feeling of trust and sharing that goes beyond what is possible through verbal communication.

  The way the music therapist engages the patient is *intentional*; the goal is to help patients realize their individual goals for healing, growth, and change. Through engagement with music, within the therapeutic relationship, a patient's abilities are strengthened and transferred to other areas of life.

**As with other forms of therapy, music therapy may be offered in a group setting.** In such cases, the music therapist engages group members in a music intervention as a way of meeting their individual goals, and the goals of the group as well.

Because a therapeutic relationship is at the heart of music therapy, it follows that listening to music by oneself, or as part of a concert audience, is not a form of music therapy, though it may be very rewarding.

- The AMTA definition proposes that music therapy involves the use of music interventions within a therapeutic relationship by "a credentialed professional who has completed an approved music therapy program." Music therapists are board certified (MT-BC). In New York State, music therapists may have a license as a creative arts therapist (LCAT).

## Broadening the definition

**As is true for other health disciplines, music therapy will continue to evolve to reflect the realities of our healthcare system—and so will our definition of music therapy.**

Today, the reality is that we don't have enough healthcare professionals in key areas. Nationally, and in certain underserved areas, we are facing a shortage of physicians, dentists, and, yes, music therapists. In response, we are learning to use our resources for the greatest good. Physicians have allocated some of their care responsibilities—quite effectively—to nurse practitioners and physician assistants (PAs). Dentists are now incorporating into their practices dental therapists—mid-level providers who can help them reach more patients in underserved areas.

Music therapists too are sharing their knowledge and skills across the healthcare team. This may involve working with nurses, recreation therapists, certified nursing assistants (CNAs), home health aides (HHAs), and musician volunteers. For example, a music therapist might share music therapy best practices with a nurse, to help her manage pain or anxiety for a patient. A music therapist might train home health aides in music therapy techniques that will enhance communication with people with dementia in their care. **Many music therapists, as clinical leaders, have come to see their role as**

**advising and training other members of the healthcare team to provide music interventions.**

This approach is yielding measurable benefits—to patients and their families, and to healthcare facilities. In music programs provided by non-music therapists, we have found that it's possible to create a safe space of caring, and acknowledge the individual in a way that creates a therapeutic relationship, if only in the moment. It is music, the shared engagement with music, that makes this happen. In Modules 5 and 6 (on dementia), we will show how caregivers who are not music therapists or musicians are using music, easily accessible online and elsewhere, to reach people with dementia in a way that can greatly enhance their experience in the present moment, and improve overall care and wellness.

## An overview of music interventions: Here's what happens
### Making music: Singing and playing musical instruments (together)

Music therapists (or recreation therapists, trained musician volunteers, or other music partners) sing and/or play music of therapeutic value to an individual patient, or a group of patients, typically on rhythm instruments, a keyboard, or guitar. They engage participants in the music, inviting them to sing or play instruments that they have provided, in line with their interests and abilities. Music therapists improvise or adjust the music to respond to individual and group needs as they emerge. Typically, they invite participants to express thoughts and emotions that are triggered by the music or the experience of music-making. The experience of music, within a therapeutic relationship, may provide opportunities for exceptional moments of human interaction.

Individuals or group members participate in:

- drumming circles; music-making with rhythm instruments (tambourines, bells, shakers, etc.), often as accompaniment to live or recorded music; music-making with melodic instruments (recorders, xylophones, guitar, electronic instruments, etc.)

- singing, one-on-one (i.e. with the music therapist), with other members of a therapeutic group, or as part of a chorus (which may include community members, caregivers, and others)

- communication of thoughts and feelings triggered by the music and music-making, with the music therapist or group leader, and with group members.

## Moving to music

The music therapist (recreation therapist, physical therapist, or occupational therapist) selects and delivers music to promote movement to meet the wellness or rehabilitation goals of participants. Music may be live or recorded.

Individuals or group members participate in:

- exercise for fitness, wellness, and falls prevention

- dance for fitness, wellness, falls prevention, and treatment of movement disorders

- movement to music as part of music-making or listening

- movement to music that is linked to (or provides cues to) specific movements, in line with rehabilitation goals (e.g. music to support range of motion exercises for stroke survivors)

- communication of thoughts and feelings triggered by the music, with the music therapist or group leader, and with group members.

## Listening to music

The music therapist or healthcare professional creates a listening experience to meet the needs of an individual (or a group), using live or recorded music. The music will reflect the musical preferences of the listener(s), and in some cases will be drawn from personalized playlists (see Module 5).

For the listening experience to be therapeutic, it must lead to a desired response. Listening to music may help a person recall memories and be more willing to share thoughts and feelings with others; or it may help a person manage anxiety and pain, feel more relaxed, or enjoy more healthful sleep. The possibilities are unlimited—and so are the settings in which listening experiences may occur. As music therapy takes place within a therapeutic relationship, it follows that the response to the listening experience should be shared with (or observed by) the music therapist or healthcare professional, to drive positive change.

Individuals or group members:

- listen to music, live or recorded

- experience and self-note responses to the listening experience; and communicate these responses to the music therapist and other healthcare professionals

- as part of a group, share listening experiences with others, communicating thoughts and exploring feelings that are triggered by the music.

An example of a streaming service is M4d Radio, available at www. imnf.org/mhp-book-resources. M4d Radio is part of the Music for Dementia Campaign to make music accessible for everyone living with dementia. It streams music from the 1930s to the 1970s, in a variety of genres, and is available all day every day, for free. The music that is streamed by M4d Radio is most likely to engage older people in general, so the service is a resource for music therapists and others who work with music listening groups across the senior care community.

## Creating music: Songwriting, composition

Music-making, as described above, provides many opportunities for participants to be creative—to make up or improvise their own music. For example, music therapists often leave out words in a song, and invite participants to fill in with words of their own; they encourage group members to improvise music that communicates their thoughts and feelings, in the moment.

In addition, music therapists may work intentionally with individuals or groups on music composition—most often songwriting. Participants in a songwriting group create words or lyrics, and compose music (or choose an existing melody) to deliver these lyrics. Most people don't have experience in creating a song, so the music therapist supports this process—technically and musically—by helping participants make choices about musical elements (such as key, tempo, dynamics), and by setting up conditions for performance or recording. A similar process supports the composition of instrumental music.

Songwriting and composition generally require leadership from music therapists or other music partners, such as musically trained staff or musician volunteers.

That said, we should note that with the explosive growth of music technology, there are limitless possibilities for people without skill or training in music to try their hand (or ear) at musical composition. Using pieces of pre-existing songs and sound, and other art media, young people have learned to express themselves creatively without relying on musical skills as traditionally defined. Similarly, when music technology is made available to older people, music composition thrives. In music therapy programs, recordings and videos can become part of the therapeutic outcome, an expression of identity, and a means of sharing oneself, and one's art, with others.

Individuals or group members:

- work with a music therapist to identify experiences and feelings that they want to convey through a song or musical composition

- engage in the composition process, with musical and technical support from the music therapist, recreation therapist, or trained musician volunteer

- share their song or musical composition with group members and others, through performance and discussion, and through recordings, videos, and other products

- explore and communicate thoughts and feelings triggered by composition and performance, with the music therapist or other music partners and group members.

## Music therapy goals (clinical goals)

Board-certified music therapists create programs and interventions that address a *broad range of goals* that are assessed and evaluated with the patient or client, and shared with the healthcare team. Below are therapeutic goals that are *representative* of the goals that music therapists can address.

### Related to sensory-motor skills

- To maintain healthy level of activity

- To increase energy, strength, and endurance in daily activities

- To improve balance and posture

- To connect to the physical responses that are stimulated by music

- To maintain and improve fine motor functioning

- To maintain and improve gross motor functioning

- To improve hand-eye coordination

- To improve visual and auditory perception

- To maintain and improve range of motion

- To improve reach-grasp-release skills

- To initiate movement in parts of the body that have limited movement

- To learn adaptive skills to compensate for temporary or permanent changes in physical function

## Related to relaxation and pain control

- To utilize relaxation and sleep inducement techniques
- To decrease and control pain (or the experience of pain)

## Related to cognitive skills

- To maintain or improve attention
- To maintain or improve short-term memory
- To improve awareness of person, place, and time
- To improve ability to count or sequence, and associate with numbers and concepts
- To improve ability to follow simple and complex directions
- To improve problem-solving

## Related to behavior in caregiving situations

- To increase participation in daily care and activities
- To increase application of on-task behaviors
- To improve ability to follow directions
- To improve awareness of self and others
- To reduce behaviors that interfere with care
- To improve ability to complete activities of daily living

## Related to communication skills

- To improve expressive language (communication of thoughts and feelings)
- To improve receptive language (ability to understand)
- To improve speech and verbal communication
- To increase effective use of nonverbal communication
- To improve communication through use of technology, including assistive technology

- To experience exceptional moments of human interaction

## Related to social skills

- To increase social interaction
- To prevent self-isolation
- To improve interpersonal skills
- To build relationships and bond to a group through shared experience
- To increase appropriate eye contact
- To increase ability to touch and be touched by others
- To increase ability to share materials and instruments with others
- To improve ability to receive feedback and constructive criticism from others
- To improve ability to give and receive praise
- To improve ability to make decisions and initiate responses
- To improve ability to appropriately interact and play with others

## Related to emotional skills

- To improve self-expression
- To improve verbal/nonverbal expression of feelings
- To improve ability to retrieve and express past/current feelings
- To improve self-esteem and achieve a heightened sense of self through proven accomplishment
- To strengthen a sense of identity
- To increase independence
- To improve coping strategies
- To improve impulse control
- To decrease stress and anxiety
- To channel feelings of anger
- To be able to express grief in times of loss
- To increase confidence that a skill can be recovered or new skill learned

- To explore spiritual awareness

- To develop creativity and explore outlets for creative expression

- To become someone other than "the patient"—"I am a musician."

### Related to professional music skills

- To learn a new skill, on a different instrument or using new technologies

- To regain a previous skill

- To retrieve a skill level that provides pleasure if not professional stature

- To learn adaptive techniques to continue to maintain enjoyment in making music

### Related to all of the above

To add a wellness piece that normalizes life within a healthcare institution.

## About benefits, risks, and outcomes

Music therapy has been shown to be effective in helping older people (and others) realize health and wellness goals, such as those listed above. These are common goals for adults of all ages, so it would seem that almost anyone can potentially benefit from music therapy, provided by a board-certified music therapist, in accordance with music therapy best practices. But "almost anyone" doesn't mean everyone—and "potentially" is no guarantee.

Not everyone benefits from music therapy as expected. That is true, of course, for most therapies: every research study that contributes to the evidence base includes subjects whose experience deviates from that of most others. With music therapy, though, there is little evidence of negative outcomes. The general understanding is that no harm will be done. *Is this true?*

In fact, music therapy is widely recognized as a safe form of therapy, without harmful side effects.

Almost all the information on music therapy that is made available to the general public focuses on positive outcomes, with no mention of risks, side effects, or contraindications. The medical community seems to be on the same page. For example, a leading hospital system with a strong institutional commitment to music therapy provides informative web pages for patients considering music therapy. In the "Benefits/Risks" section, no risks are mentioned.

Experienced music therapists and clinicians at that top-tier hospital can conceive of cases where music therapy presents risks to an individual patient, or results in harmful side effects. These cases are so rare, *and the risks so easily anticipated*, that cautionary words seem unnecessary for those seeking everyday guidance. What's more, the harmful side effects that occur in music therapy are not life threatening, and do not significantly affect a patient's long-term function or mortality.

Here are examples of risks associated with music therapy for patients in a senior care environment, as identified by the IMNF, over 25 years of experience.

- Certain tone frequencies or strong rhythmic patterns in music can trigger seizures in vulnerable patients, such as people with certain forms of epilepsy (e.g. temporal lobe epilepsy). Such reactions are very rare and do not have long-term effects.

- For people with frontal temporal dementia, music can sound like horrible noise or static. Frontal temporal dementia affects the temporal lobes in the brain. The right temporal lobe is responsible for processing the actual tones in music. When this area is damaged the person may no longer hear any tones in music and consequently no longer hears a melody. Only about 10–20 percent of people with dementia are diagnosed with frontal temporal dementia (and the majority of these patients are younger than the dementia population as a whole). Music therapists, in practice, assess for these issues, so negative responses are rare.

- A song that is associated with a traumatic experience can trigger depression or emotional withdrawal. In most cases, this is addressed and resolved in one or more music therapy sessions. Sometimes, though, the depression is severe, leading to profound withdrawal or other negative outcomes. For an example of how this can occur, we draw from experience with a music listening group (which was not at that time part of a music therapy program): on admission to a nursing home, a resident was referred to an "opera club" because she enjoyed classical music. The group chose to listen to an opera by Wagner. On hearing the opening notes of "The Ride of the Valkyries," the new resident gasped and collapsed. She remained nonverbal for more than a week. She had been in a concentration camp where this music had been played.

  Music can trigger powerful emotions, including negative and debilitating emotions. This is a reality that music therapists take into account and are qualified to address with a patient or client. But when severe responses happen unexpectedly, and are not well resolved, we must recognize a harmful side effect of music therapy.

Although it is rare that a music therapist or administrator of a senior care agency might report an adverse event due to music therapy practice, it is critically important to acknowledge the risks that are identified, and any harmful side effects that occur.

## The Sound Health Initiative

*Although the health benefits of music therapy are widely recognized, music therapy is not widely available throughout the US healthcare system. This is about to change...*

In 2019, the National Institutes of Health (NIH) awarded $20 million over five years to explore the benefits of music on health. Initial research will support the Sound Health Initiative, which will focus on understanding music's mechanisms of action in the brain, and how this understanding may be applied, clinically, to treat Parkinson's disease, stroke, chronic pain, and other neurological disorders.

The NIH, which represents the interests of all of us, has committed our medical and research institutions to support research into music therapy, so as to explore, *and make widely available*, the benefits of music therapy that we identify. This commitment was made because it is widely believed, on the basis of medical evidence, that the benefits of music therapy are significant. And with emerging brain science, we have new understanding and technologies to collect the evidence. The Sound Health Initiative is an NIH-Kennedy Center for the Performing Arts partnership in association with the National Endowment for the Arts.

To learn more about the Sound Health Initiative, visit www.imnf.org/mhp-book-resources.

# An Introduction to Music Interventions: The Therapeutic Drumming Circle

One way to learn about music therapy is to observe or participate in a music intervention.

Thanks to YouTube and training videos, it is possible to view music therapists online as they demonstrate therapeutic uses of music in different settings, with different populations. In-person observation is even better. If you work in a setting where music therapists are part of the healthcare team, you may be able to observe music interventions, in real time, as part of treatment and care.

Perhaps the best way to come to an understanding of music therapy is to participate in a music intervention and experience the therapeutic benefits yourself. For this reason, we have chosen to introduce music therapy through therapeutic drumming circles, a music intervention in which nearly everyone can participate.

Therapeutic drumming has been shown to be one of the most effective tools we have for creating a sense of community among people with dementia. It's also a powerful way of relieving depression and anxiety in people of all ages. Most importantly, therapeutic drumming circles are inclusive experiences, with the potential to address the wellness needs of everyone in a community. In a skilled nursing facility or senior residence, therapeutic drumming circles often include CNAs, administrators, and family members, along with residents or patients.

## What happens in a therapeutic drumming circle?

In a therapeutic drumming session, participants meet in a circle, and each is given (or selects) a simple rhythm instrument, such as a hand drum, frame drum, tambourine, or maracas. **The circle establishes a feeling of inclusion** and belonging: there is no hierarchy of staff and patient, of well and unwell; everyone's contribution is equally important, and equally valued.

The leader (or co-leaders) of the drumming circle stand or sit where they can see and be easily seen by all members. They will give many visual cues in the course of the drumming, and may move around the circle, and among participants. The leader(s) may be assisted by one or more facilitators who demonstrate the action and reinforce the rhythm.

**Therapeutic drumming is based on the fact that people are psychologically and neurologically primed to respond to a regular beat.** The leader establishes a simple rhythm with a strong beat. The usual way to do this is to accent the first beat (also called the downbeat) in a group of three or four beats (a musical measure)—1-2-3, 1-2-3, 1-2-3, and so on; or 1-2-3-4, 1-2-3-4, 1-2-3-4, and so on.

To begin the group, the leader establishes the rhythm and goes around the circle, welcoming each member by name, *in rhythm*. The leader will typically chant words such as "hello, hello" and "what is your name?" to a rhythm and melody that become the basis for an exchange with other group members.

To view a "Welcome" sequence from an IMNF therapeutic drumming circle for people with dementia and their caregivers, visit www.imnf.org/mhp-book-resources.

In the course of the session, leaders typically improvise, or vary the drumming, to engage the group, in line with therapeutic purposes. The drumming may become a "call and response" exercise, in which group members echo the leader's beat. A chant may be added, or improvised. The leader may vary the dynamics (signaling when to play loud or soft); they may introduce pauses and other variations that command attention and focus. When the group has been playing together for a while, the leader may call for solos from group members. In every case, the leader will give verbal and visual cues to keep the group together, in the moment, and in rhythm.

To view a later sequence from the IMNF therapeutic drumming circle for people with dementia and their caregivers, visit www.imnf.org/mhp-book-resources.

The therapeutic drumming session will typically close with a winding-down exercise, such as a goodbye chant or song, or a rousing "call and response" that calls the session to end. Because therapeutic drumming is an expressive activity, and often an emotional experience, group members may continue to interact and share their feelings after the session has ended.

Note that while we have described a model of the therapeutic drumming circle, there are many variations on this model, reflecting the needs and preferences of different communities.

## What does therapeutic drumming tell us about music interventions in general?

### 1. Therapeutic drumming is a rhythmic activity

> Most of the music interventions that you will encounter in this guidebook are rhythmic activities.

A rhythmic activity is any activity in which people respond to a strong and steady musical beat, for example by moving or making sounds in time with the beat.

Rhythmic activities include movements such as drumming, clapping, walking, and dancing in time to a musical beat, as well as singing, chanting, playing musical instruments, and many other activities. Even listening can be a rhythmic activity: you may feel the beat as you listen, even if you don't tap your foot or nod your head in time to the music (though probably you will).

### 2. Therapeutic drumming is...therapeutic!

> All music interventions have a therapeutic purpose or goal—in health and wellness, in treatment and rehabilitation.

What makes a rhythmic activity therapeutic is that it is a shared experience with a therapeutic purpose. In the therapeutic drumming circle, many goals or therapeutic outcomes are possible for individuals and for the group itself. Mickey Hart, the Grateful Dead drummer (and founder of the wellness organization "Rhythm for Life"), has described the potential effects of drumming on older people in congregate settings:

First, there would be immediate reduction in feelings of loneliness and alienation through interaction with each other and heightened contact with the outside world... Whereas verbal communication can often be difficult...in the drum circle nonverbal communication is the means of relating. Natural byproducts of this are increased self-esteem and the resulting sense of empowerment, creativity, and enhanced ability to focus the mind, not to mention just plain fun.

This leads to a reduction in stress, while involving the body in a non-jarring, safe form of exercise that invigorates, energizes, and centers. (Hart, 1991)

Note that therapeutic drumming addresses basic human needs, such as the need for belongingness and communication, as well as what we sometimes consider to be higher needs, such as the need for self-esteem and creativity. Physical needs are also addressed: participating in a therapeutic drumming circle may result in a reduction of tension, an increase in energy or mobility, and better circulation and respiration. (And there is some evidence that drumming may also bolster the immune system.) Cognitive benefits may include an increased ability to focus, follow instructions, and attend to tasks at hand. Most music interventions have the potential to meet needs, and achieve positive outcomes, in more than one area of health and wellness.

Because the therapeutic drumming circle focuses on therapeutic outcomes, *participants don't need to worry about meeting performance standards.* We know from experience that many people are nervous about participating in a new activity, due to embarrassment or fears of failure. But *in music interventions, participation, at any level, is celebrated.* Participants in a therapeutic drumming circle can come in and out of the drumming at their own pace, without feeling that they must apologize for "mistakes." As in other music interventions, it's not about performance—except in that performing is meaningful and therapeutic to the person.

### 3. Therapeutic drumming circles are inclusive and accessible to almost everyone

In general, music interventions do not require music training and experience on the part of participants. Rhythmic activities, as well as most other music interventions, can be adapted to meet the needs of people at all levels of functioning.

Participants in a therapeutic drumming circle do not need to have had music experience. They don't need to speak a given language, or to be able to speak at all. They don't have to demonstrate any level of cognitive and physical function, or mental health status. In fact, people living with late-stage dementia often participate vigorously in drumming circles. People who are unable to hold drumsticks can participate by stamping their feet or using foot pedals. And people who are depressed, withdrawn, or isolated are among the most likely to benefit in this expressive group activity.

Therapeutic drumming circles and other rhythmic activities are very well suited for mixed or culturally diverse populations—one reason that they have evolved into community events. In skilled nursing communities, the IMNF has conducted therapeutic drumming circles that include residents in all stages of dementia, as well as higher functioning residents, CNAs, and nursing and administrative staff. This, it has been shown, works well: the IMNF model for dementia-inclusive drumming has been disseminated widely, with support from the New York State Department of Health (Tomaino *et al.*, 2008).

### Amplification

*Although we've said that you don't need to have music experience to participate in music interventions,* there are seniors in care who are (or have been) professional or amateur musicians. For those who might want to return to an instrument or vocal repertoire, music therapists can offer therapeutic interventions that are keyed to their music abilities and goals. In addition, experience shows that musician volunteers and music specialists are able (with training) to make music, and compose and improvise music, with people in care settings. But the focus here, as in all music interventions, is therapeutic: for example, the goal for a musician in senior care might be to retrieve a musical skill that gives pleasure, to improve self-esteem, or to have opportunities for meaningful interactions with the music therapist and other music lovers.

## 4. Therapeutic drumming is a form of nonverbal communication

Like music itself, music interventions are nonverbal communications; they have the power to move us, without words or language. Music interventions rely on rhythm, melody, and other elements of music, to get through to us in ways that words, alone, do not.

In a therapeutic drumming circle, feelings are expressed and communicated through drumming itself—through vibrations and sounds that are perceived as rhythm and music. Words are not necessary, which is to say that drumming is a form of *nonverbal communication*.

Why is this important? We know from experience that rhythm—a beat—can move us (make us move). *What we learn in the drumming circle is that rhythm can enable us to communicate with one another, and create a group experience with a particular outcome.* Like the hand-clapping of the kindergarten teacher, or the drum beats of a marching band, therapeutic drumming tells people how to move together, and be together. Like the pulsing of disco music in a club, the drumming tells everyone in the group how others are moving, and why, and in what spirit.

**As we will see, part of the reason that music interventions are so powerful is that *they don't rely on the usual mechanisms of verbal communication.* No one tells people in the drumming circle to move together—it just happens. Language seems to have little to do with this. With people with dementia, for example, we often say that "music gets through when words do not." This is true, in fact, for all of us.**

Music and other forms of nonverbal communication, such as "body language," are processed in parts of the brain that are shared with verbal language. These nonverbal messages play an important role—much larger than we realize—in our experience of the world. For people who find it difficult or impossible to communicate with words—due to depression or dementia, for example—nonverbal communications, especially music, become vitally important. In this guidebook, we will discover many healthcare situations in which music interventions provide meaningful sound when communication skills have deteriorated.

### Amplification

Although therapeutic drumming and other rhythmic activities are a form of nonverbal communication, that doesn't mean that words have no part in these activities. The leader of the drumming circle will call out names or encouragements, such as "Go, Martha, go!" or "How high can we go?" He may incorporate song phrases, or refrains, or make up chants that resonate with group members. Even so, the music intervention retains the characteristics of a nonverbal communication: words chanted or sung to music get through to us through the power of music.

**Brain science tells us that when words are embedded in music, they are processed in a way that is quite different from the way we process ordinary speech.** Parents and teachers know this intuitively: they use sing-song with young children to convey information, encouragement, or instruction, knowing that the child probably wouldn't get the message if addressed in a speaking tone. Try saying "You need to wash your hands and here's how... " compared to "This is the way we wash our hands, wash our hands, wash our hands..." The music and accompanying movement—the nonverbal elements—convey the message more effectively than words to a person (in this case a small child) who does not have full language or attention capabilities. So it is for us, always, in our lives, and especially when words fail.

This is not surprising (if you think of it). The rhythm and melody of speech (the way we raise or lower our voices) impart essential meanings to ordinary speech. This helps explain why children who have language delays often have problems in rhythm perception as well; they are deficient in the ability to understand sound patterns that underlie both speech and music (Ladányi *et al.*, 2020).

Drumming and other rhythmic activities communicate through rhythmic patterns and their variations. Other music interventions that we will encounter use songs, or words embedded in familiar music, to communicate with people, and help them reach their therapeutic goals.

## 5. The therapeutic drumming circle takes place in a social context—it is in part a social activity

Participation in therapeutic drumming has the potential to increase the social engagement and well-being of group members.

> One could say, as some researchers do, that all music-making is social, that all music takes place in a social context (MacDonald, 2013; Brancatisano *et al.*, 2020).

What we know is that music interventions, when successful, almost always have positive effects on social (or psychosocial) well-being. This is true of interventions that explicitly target socialization, such as groups for people with depression or dementia—and also for interventions that target movement and speech disorders.

At the most basic level, music groups (both recreational and therapeutic) bring people together, to interact around a shared activity. Among older people in congregate settings, such group activities are an important defense against social isolation and loneliness, which are known to contribute to physical and mental decline. Music interventions are effective in addressing social needs in this population because of the unique attributes of music, as described above. For example, participants can interact with others around music-making, singing, or listening, even when speech and communication skills have deteriorated; they can move together—and perhaps bond with one another—without needing to respond to verbal direction or other cognitive demands. In addition, participation in a music group often leads to a more positive mood, and better relationships between group members.

Group music interventions can be especially helpful to people who are recovering from stroke or living with a progressive neurological disease, such as dementia or Parkinson's disease. For these individuals, loss of function too often results in loss of meaningful social activities, leading to a loss of confidence and social identity—and sometimes to depression. Group music interventions provide opportunities to explore these feelings through music, and shared responses to music; a main focus of this group work is to restore the feeling of "belongingness" that is essential to well-being.

In this guidebook, we will describe group music interventions, focusing on specific techniques that have positive effects on social engagement for people with a range of healthcare needs. At the same time, we should note that social interaction takes place outside the group framework—for example, between a music therapist and patient in an individual session; and between a CNA or HHA and patient during everyday care. These interventions too have the potential to improve social engagement and well-being.

### 6. The basic techniques of therapeutic drumming can by mastered by staff who are not music therapists or music specialists

> Music therapists have established best practices that are based on years of clinical experience and research. In many cases, these best practices can be generalized for use by other members of the health-care team, and by trained volunteers, including musician volunteers.

In this guidebook, we will present music interventions that involve techniques that are accessible to people who are not music therapists or music specialists. Therapeutic drumming is just one example of a "tried and true" intervention that can be delivered by a broad cast of well-trained staff members and volunteers. Other music interventions may require collaboration between music therapists and specific healthcare professionals. For example, rehabilitation for stroke survivors may involve music therapists working in partnership with speech and language pathologists, physical therapists, and occupational therapists.

In a therapeutic drumming circle, the leader may be a music therapist who is assisted by two facilitators—for example, a recreation therapist and a CNA who has been trained in delivering rhythmic activities (or has experience as a drumming circle participant). In other cases, the leader may be a recreation therapist or CNA who has mastered basic practices of therapeutic drumming through participation in a workshop or certification program. Musician volunteers, percussionists, and others can also be leaders and facilitators.

For senior care communities, having a music therapy department or music therapist on site increases the possibilities for delivering music interventions across the community. Staff who are not music therapists will benefit from ongoing opportunities to learn from music therapists to apply best practices, within the scope of their own practice and abilities.

## 7. Participation in therapeutic drumming activities has real and measurable benefits to frontline caregivers, to other staff members in a senior care community, and to the community itself

> Music interventions have the potential to be therapeutic for caregivers as well as for the people in their care.

The therapeutic drumming circle is an example of a music intervention that integrates staff members with those who are usually called "patients" or "residents." CNAs join the drumming circle, and participate alongside people with dementia and other challenges—*the same people who usually require their care.*

Research suggests that when staff and "patients" or "residents" come together as equal partners in music-making, they are able to see one another as "real people." This enhances person-centered care, and the sense of community.

For caregiving staff, as for others, the therapeutic drumming circle is an opportunity to share a pleasurable experience in an atmosphere of mutually successful participation. And it's fun!

> In this video, you see caregiver and patient interaction during the "wind down" of a therapeutic drumming circle. The participants have turned in their instruments, and are preparing to go forward to the next part of their day: www.imnf.org/mhp-book-resources.

One study of caregivers' experiences noted that "music therapeutic caregiving" (their term) led to communication being "mutually awakened," for people with dementia. This resulted in "feelings of happiness" and "feelings of well-being" in the caregivers, which seem to have been communicated to their patients with dementia. As one caregiver said, "when you are working with someone that is always stressed out and sad you get stressed out yourself, but when I am singing that is not the case anymore...the situation is nice, and it is fun to do" (Hammar *et al.*, 2010). IMNF programs that have used videos to assist caregivers in music-making activities with people with dementia have been shown to increase caregiver satisfaction, confidence, and morale.

## Therapeutic drumming: "It's the number one interdisciplinary team vitamin!"

Some years ago the IMNF received funding from the New York State Department of Health (NYSDOH), to train staff at four "consortium nursing homes" to initiate and sustain therapeutic drumming circles and other rhythm-based activities as a regular part of the therapeutic recreation program provided to residents living with dementia (Tomaino *et al.*, 2008). This large project, completed in 2008, led to other IMNF initiatives that involved staff training in rhythmic activities, with evaluation of outcomes for both patients and staff.

Reports from the original consortium nursing homes showed that therapeutic rhythm and drumming programs had many positive effects on staff well-being. "It's the number one interdisciplinary team vitamin!" was one response.

Comments touched on the following points:

- The support of administration is vital when implementing a new program such as therapeutic drumming.

- Therapeutic rhythm and drumming programs elicit support from administration, as they see and understand the therapeutic benefits of rhythmic activities for residents with dementia.

- Rhythmic activities bring staff closer while emphasizing the concept of teamwork and leadership.

- Staff understand that they don't have to be professionally trained percussionists or musicians to take part in or lead a therapeutic rhythm program; thus more are taking part in and leading these programs.

- When caregivers are participating in or leading the activities, as opposed to merely being observers, the residents' responses are increased and intensified.

- Implementing a rhythm program strengthens the feeling of community throughout the facility.

- Therapeutic rhythm activities have the capacity to reach a wide range of participants, from very low-functioning residents, to high-functioning family members and friends.

- Many residents are from different cultural backgrounds and rhythm is able to reach residents of all cultures since it does not rely solely on language.

- The rhythm activities integrate the cultural backgrounds of the staff with the cultural backgrounds of the patients.

- Rhythmic activities allow for the age barrier between staff and residents to diminish, and even disappear.

- Drumming activities unite the community of residents and staff, strengthening the interdisciplinary team, and giving the opportunity for optimal well-being of residents, staff, family members, and visitors.

---

The IMNF has at times offered therapeutic drumming circles *specifically* for caregiving staff. Therapeutic goals for staff might include the following:

- Reducing levels of stress and anxiety.

- Increasing energy through physical exercise and sensory stimulation.

- Improving mood and sense of well-being.

- Enhancing creativity and self-esteem in the caregiving role and generally.

- Strengthening relationships with staff colleagues.

**Addendum:** We began with an introduction to music interventions with the therapeutic drumming circle, because this is an activity that is therapeutic, and fun, for everyone. You might wonder if there are other ways for staff members and people in the community to participate in therapeutic music-making, along with seniors in their care. And there are.

Choruses made up of people with dementia and their caregivers are popping up in the US, and in Australia, Canada, and the UK. It's a growing trend. The choruses are mostly community-based groups, serving people with mild to moderate dementia and their family caregivers. But the model has potential for senior care settings, and for seniors at all levels of functioning (see Module 5).

Also of interest are instrumental groups made up of community musicians and people in senior care who are professional or amateur musicians. Creating such groups involves careful preparation, and an understanding of each participant's abilities; but isn't that the case for any music ensemble? Or any creative project?

Therapeutic drumming circles, choruses, and instrumental ensembles offer new ways of integrating seniors in care with the larger community. Everyone benefits: individual seniors, their family care partners (who often feel painfully isolated), professional caregivers across senior care settings, and the community itself. Choruses and instrumental groups that develop out of these music interventions often give performances (a few even go on tour). The goal is to bring to others the joy of music, along with an awareness of the potential for everyone, including those with dementia, to be part of, and continue to contribute to, the community.

## How to mount a therapeutic drumming circle in your senior care community
### The basics
#### Goals

As a first step, the healthcare team that is responsible for planning the therapeutic drumming circle will meet to discuss general goals for participants and for the group as a whole. For example, goals might include: to improve mood or sense of well-being; to create feelings of community and belonging; to increase social interaction and communication between staff and patients—whatever goals reflect the needs of the intended participants.

#### The leader: What to look for

A critical step in mounting a therapeutic drumming circle is to identify a well-qualified leader.

The leader should be a music therapist, or a person who has received training from a music therapist, for example in a workshop or in-service training that reflects the best practices of music therapy. The training experience should also include *practice* under the guidance of a music therapist or other qualified mentor. Leaders will seek to create a shared experience with a therapeutic purpose. They must be able to energize and inspire others. And most importantly, they must be able to observe and respond to participants in a way that helps them reach their goals, which might be social goals, or rehabilitation goals, for example.

Here are the main skills or competencies you will need in a leader of a therapeutic drumming circle:

- The leader must be able to maintain control of the rhythm (the beat) at all times. This requires more experience than one might imagine. Establishing a strong and steady beat is not difficult. But leaders must maintain the beat as a constant in all interactions with participants. They must not lose the beat if participants do not respond as expected—if they do not call out their name, for example, in a greeting exercise. Instead, the leader will repeat the rhythm, and give the participant another chance; or they will call out the name (if they know it), or perhaps say something like "Go, go, my friend," and move on, *in rhythm*, to the next participant. Similarly, if an instrument clatters to the floor, or some other distraction occurs, the leader will respond to this rhythmically—that is, within the rhythm established—because it is rhythm that makes possible the shared experience, and the therapeutic outcome.

- Leaders will know how to improvise, or creatively alter the music, as they interact with the group and individual members. As an example, a leader might increase/decrease the tempo (or speed) at which the rhythm is driven to intensify engagement, or slow the tempo to wind down. In the video sequences included here we see improvisations involving dynamics, rhythmic chants, verbal call-outs, and much more. It is important that leaders know how and *when* to initiate the improvisation; for example, *when it will be therapeutic* to intensify engagement. Improvisation plays an essential role in therapeutic music activities; and so group leaders, in general, should be familiar and comfortable with the basics of improvisation.

- Facilitators are participants who assist the leader. Especially in large groups, it is helpful if two or more staff members can serve as facilitators. As the leader gives visual and verbal cues, facilitators who are positioned around the circle can model these cues up close to participants, and provide other support. It's worth noting that recruiting facilitators may help your institution train staff members to lead rhythmic activities, including future therapeutic drumming circles.

Downloadable HANDOUT at www.imnf.org/mhp-book-resources.

# How to lead a therapeutic drumming circle: Tips and techniques

*Marlon Sobol, MT-BC, LCAT, staff music therapist,*
*IMNF project, "Rhythmic Activities for Everyday Care"*

## When you're the leader...

- Smile, introduce self, get everybody feeling comfortable and relaxed but on the edge.

- Assure the group, "You don't have to ever have played drums before to participate in a drum circle."

## Techniques you can use

- **Thunder rolls:** Rolling from the middle to edge of the drum. Getting acquainted with the drum.

- **The 1-2-3 beat:** Also known as: "We will rock you" beat. (You don't have to sing the song.) Get everybody playing in time. Follow low tones.

- **Visual cues:** The more animated the better. Move while you play so people have something to visually follow.

- **Split up parts:** One half of the group gets beats 1–2, the other half gets 3. Then switch around. For example, with the James Brown song "Hit Me," everybody plays however many hits the leader calls out. ("Hit me twice," "Hit me three times," etc.)

- **Call and response:** The leader plays a phrase and the group repeats the same phrase or the leader plays a phrase and the group finishes it.

- **Melody fill-in:** The leader sings melody, the group finishes phrase.

- **Solos:** The leader calls out a name of a person to take a solo. The soloist passes it on to another group member. The leader provides lots of positive reinforcement and encourages group members to take advantage of the moment where they can "shine" individually.

- **Group follows beat of soloist:** The soloist starts soloing and then begins a beat where the group follows. If the beat is strong, go with it. If the beat is not strong, fade it out to the next soloist.

- **Sing song with a beat:** The leader sings a simple song, something everybody can relate to, easy to sing along with, inspiring, with a universal message. Chants are always successful—as melodies without lyrics, or melodies with repetitive lyrics. Chants can be created on simple phrases relevant with group members: for example, "I am strong," "I will beat my pain away."

- **Close session:** Thank the group for creating this experience together and allowing the leader to be a part of it. Leave group feeling empowered and inter-dependent. *Not independent* and *not dependent* but *inter-dependent*.

### Time requirements

A therapeutic drumming circle session will usually last about an hour, with 15 minutes for set-up, and 45 minutes for the drumming activity. Shorter sessions are also a possibility.

### Participants

Anyone is welcome in a community therapeutic drumming circle. In a senior care setting, this might include administrators, health professionals at all levels, frontline caregivers, dieticians and kitchen staff, and so on, as well as people in care or assisted living.

How do we engage staff in this activity? Recruitment of staff to participate in a therapeutic drumming circle can be part of a larger initiative that educates staff about music therapy, and creates excitement around music programming in the community.

Promotion and education should be part of the set-up. Flyers, electronic communications, web postings, or other internal communications can be used to present therapeutic drumming as a pleasurable activity with positive outcomes.

Participation of residents and patients will likely come through referrals from staff, or as self-referrals from people in assisted or independent living. People at all levels of functioning can be encouraged to participate, even those with moderate-to-severe dementia, and those who have little to no motor activity.

For people with serious physical issues, it is often possible to create *adaptive instruments*. For example, staff can attach Velcro to bells or mallets and affix them to a person's hands or shoes. This allows someone with limited fine motor skills to participate in rhythmic music-making. Creating adaptive instruments usually requires advance preparation, though. Other options are to welcome people with physical limitations, and ask them to nod, tap, or move to the beat.

For people who are sound-sensitive, including those with dementia who may become overly aroused by loud drum sounds, a softer and more therapeutic drum sound may be achieved with a REMO drumhead using Comfort Sound Drum Technology®.

Group size can range from 3 to 30 (or more) participants. For larger groups, it is recommended to have at least one facilitator to assist the leader (and/or co-leaders).

Although the community therapeutic drumming circle will welcome adults of all ages and levels of function, healthcare facilities may offer therapeutic drumming for specific populations, for example for people with dementia, or for people on a specific living unit. The size of the drumming circle will vary accordingly.

### Materials

Practically any rhythm instrument can be used in a therapeutic drumming circle. Below is a sample list of instruments that are handy to have on hand for drumming as well as other music interventions. Note that with the exception of a few drums, none of these instruments is essential for a drumming circle. While it's great to be able to offer participants a wide selection of instruments, you can generally use whatever is at hand. (That's because virtually anything we touch can make rhythm.) Simple percussion instruments are inexpensive (in many cases under $20). Some, like shakers and rhythm sticks, you can make from materials at hand. But be mindful of sound quality. Drums should be of good sound quality: they can cost from $30 to $150.

### Drums

| | |
|---|---|
| Paddle drums with holders | Frame drums |
| Floor drums | Djembe drums |
| Hand drums | Tubanos |

### Other rhythm instruments

| | |
|---|---|
| Maracas | Mallets (pair) |
| Tambourines | Wrist bells |
| Claves | Cow bells |
| Rhythm sticks | Agogo bells |

| | |
|---|---|
| Finger cymbals | Shakers |
| Woodblocks | Xylophone |
| Guiros | |

## Physical environment and equipment requirements

A therapeutic drumming circle requires minimal preparation. In most cases you will need:

- a large open area with chairs in a circle. This area should not be adjacent to any rooms or passageways that require quiet at the time the activity will take place

- instruments attractively displayed for selection

- a swivel chair for the leader, if possible

- a headset microphone for the leader

- an amplifier for the microphone or for recorded music

- if recorded music is used, an iPad or MP3 player, and so on

- for community events, if appropriate, a small welcome table, with sign-in sheets, handouts, and so on.

## Feedback and evaluation

On completion of the therapeutic drumming circle, the healthcare team will want to solicit feedback from participants, including administrative and clinical staff who will be involved in shaping and evaluating future programs. A simple post-activity survey might be distributed to participants who are able and willing to complete it.

> To access sample downloadable evaluation forms for therapeutic drumming circles and other therapeutic rhythm-based activities that may be offered to your patient population, visit www.imnf.org/mhp-book-resources.

For those with dementia or other cognitive or motor difficulties, a survey may be developed to encourage staff and family care partners to record their observations of the effect of the activity on the person (or persons) in their care.

- The post-activity survey might include open-ended questions, such as *"Please summarize your experience today in the drumming circle."* This might be followed by prompts; for example, *"Describe any changes you noticed in your energy level, mood, motor skills, and so on after participating in the drumming. Describe any new skills that you learned."*

- Short-answer questions might focus on the goals of the activity. For example, *"After participating in today's drumming circle I felt a greater sense of belonging and community."* (Rate: 1=strongly disagree, 2=disagree, 3=agree, 4=strongly agree, 0=not sure.)

- An important question is *"How likely are you to participate in another drumming circle, if one is offered?"* or *"How likely are you to recommend that your patient(s) participate in another drumming circle if one is offered?"* (Rate: 1=very likely, 2=likely, 3=somewhat likely, 4=not likely.)

- Results of the survey, as well as other feedback, should be shared with the leader(s) and facilitators; in turn, leaders might be asked to submit their own evaluation of the drumming circle, citing highlights and noting what worked well and not so well (and "lessons learned").

## A personal note to colleagues in music therapy, and colleagues in senior healthcare

I have been encouraged for a very long time to put together this best practice guide on the use of music in senior wellness and healthcare. I've been immersed in the work for so long—and have been joined by so many other voices—that sometimes I think that what I have to say is already common knowledge. So I asked myself, who needs this book? Who can benefit from these best practices that music therapists know are effective in enhancing wellness and improving function for the seniors in our care?

Music therapy as a health profession has grown tremendously over the last 20 years. There are now excellent guides, as well as numerous journal articles by music therapists and other researchers, which provide guidance on the benefits of music in senior care. But still I hear from so many people who believe they have "discovered" how beneficial music is in caring for a family member, how music makes a loved one (thought to be irretrievably submerged in dementia) come alive, at home or in the course of a nursing home visit. The many people who contact me usually want more information on what they should do right now, and why, and how. I have come to realize that there is a real need to provide clearer guidance, with examples, that will enable more people to use music in everyday care.

Recent media coverage of iconic singers like Glen Campbell and Tony

Bennett, both of whom could perform and take pleasure from their music despite advanced Alzheimer's disease, has increased public awareness of the importance of music in memory care. Now the challenge is how to make music therapy-informed programs more accessible in healthcare facilities and at home. So how do we do this?

Although I think that every healthcare agency should have a music therapist on staff, the reality is that those agencies that provide music therapy are usually served by a music therapist who visits once or twice a week for special group programs. Such programs only touch the surface of what is needed. The relatively few music therapists who work full time in senior care agencies often share responsibilities with therapeutic recreation and are unable to provide the intensive clinical work that would have the biggest impact, especially in areas of behavioral health and subacute rehabilitation. What works best, I've found, is for the music therapist to partner with and train other team members, including direct care staff and volunteers, who can then use music effectively in everyday care, and also in rehabilitation.

It's easy to see why music therapists need partners on the ground in senior care. According to the Centers for Disease Control and Prevention (CDC), there were 15,600 nursing homes in the US (in 2016), providing care to 1.3 million current residents (in 2015); and a total of 4.5 million patients received or ended care during the year 2015 (Sengupta et al., 2022). Even with the number of professional board-certified music therapists increasing every year—presently at about 10,000—only a small percentage work in senior care, and those who do often work on a per diem basis. We are left to imagine what would be possible with better integrated music therapy and music-informed programs.

A fundamental challenge is funding: most senior care facilities operate on a capitated rate per resident, meaning that there are no funds for anything more than basic, essential services. There may be one certified therapeutic recreation specialist (which is the standard requirement for patient care charting) who oversees activity programs. Special programs like music therapy are often funded by donors and grants. These programs are born in enthusiasm and commitment, and often result in measurable benefits for patients (and the institution itself). But funders tend to focus on their special interests—on specific patient groups, for example—and few funders can commit to sustainability. So, again, we are not in a position to achieve what would be possible with well-integrated music therapy and music-informed programs across the community.

The bright spot is that there have been efforts to train direct care staff to use music in a more purposeful way. The challenge is that this training is not likely to be reinforced at the agency level—not without greater efforts on our part. The training of staff in music therapy best practices, to be effective, must involve education and dialogue with healthcare leaders and administrators across the organization. That is something we are working on, in the profession, and in this guidebook.

Another bright spot is that many healthcare facilities now welcome musicians (and other performing artists) to the care environment. There are professional music organizations and individual musicians who would like to do more than just entertain. But again, there are challenges: we sometimes see push-back or reluctance by music therapists, due to lack of time or resources, when it comes to training others to use music with therapeutic intent; and there are concerns about potential competition for paid music therapy opportunities, because there are scarce opportunities, after all.

*But this may be changing...*

Currently a national effort is underway to expand the role of arts in all aspects of healthcare. This has helped focus attention on important questions about efficacy, funding, and oversight. I believe there is a leadership role for music therapists—as clinicians, researchers, and advocates—in the "arts in healthcare" initiatives that are now before us. As music therapists, working on the ground, we can have an advisory role to senior care communities that are exploring ways to use music therapeutically, in skilled nursing homes, home care, subacute rehab, assisted living, and independent living units. We can also lead efforts to help develop a national strategy for training musician volunteers to provide therapeutic music experiences to seniors and their care partners.

I believe that there is enough evidence of the benefits of music—to soothe, reduce pain, improve mood, and improve and connect memories—that some of these therapeutic uses of music should be considered similar to over-the-counter medications; that is, taken for likely benefit, with some guidance and precaution, but generally with little potential harm.

In other words, a music therapy intervention, such as the use of familiar songs with people with dementia, might be delivered by trained, informed caregiving staff, or musician volunteers, with music therapists looking on. I can say this, with confidence, because I have overseen outstanding therapeutic work from music therapy students, from trained musician volunteers, from trained direct care staff, and from social workers and other healthcare professionals who happen to have music backgrounds. As in medical practice, if a situation needs more than an over-the-counter approach, as would be the case for someone with a mental illness or complex health problem, then a music therapist should be consulted.

This guidebook aims to consolidate more than 40 years of music therapy practices that have come through the Institute for Music and Neurologic Function. It is our hope that, for other agencies, and the field in general, this guidebook will provide a framework for training programs that incorporate the best practices of the IMNF and others. Another aim in providing this guide is to share with senior care administrators the benefits of music therapy and informed music programming, so as to enlist their expertise and advocacy in training direct care staff to use music with intent when providing for those in their care.

MODULE 3

# Getting Started: Bringing Music Therapy Best Practices to Your Organization

In many homes, listening to music, or making music, is a shared activity. So it is not surprising that many family caregivers have discovered, on their own, the power of music in caring for a loved one. And they want to know more.

Training in music therapy best practices empowers these family caregivers, and professional caregivers as well. The experience of a caregiver who participated in the Canadian "Music Care" training program is instructive—and inspiriting.

> Before I began the music care training, I thought I knew a lot about the benefits of music. I had been singing to my mom for years, who has advanced Alzheimer's disease, and have seen how beneficial the music was. I was amazed at how much I did not know and to learn how powerful a tool music is and the many ways it can be used. For example, how music and humming can have a calming effect; how ascending and descending melodies have different effects and how music can evoke memories and reduce depression and loneliness. (Foster *et al.*, 2021, p.11)

The therapeutic effects of music have long been recognized by those who care for loved ones at home, or for patients in senior care communities. And never more so than today.

The media and social media are alive with videos, personal accounts, and scientific studies about how powerful a tool music is and how it can be used. **The inevitable result is that more and more people want access to music therapy, to support their health and wellness goals and to help them care for loved ones. In many cases, the need is urgent.**

And here's the challenge. Music therapy is NOT readily accessible through our healthcare system, due to a lack of both music therapy providers and a reliable system to deliver the service to those who would benefit. Where music therapy is available, it is seldom covered by insurance, which means that it is not accessible to people of ordinary means, in ordinary circumstances. These are broad challenges that we cannot fully address here.

Our focus is on senior care settings, and here we are seeing progress:

- Increasingly, music therapists are sharing their skills with other members of the healthcare team. Recreation therapists, certified nursing assistants, and home health aides are being trained to provide music interventions within their scope of practice and music experience. Music therapists are also sharing their skills with family care partners, directly, at healthcare facilities, and by partnering with nonprofit organizations that provide information and training to caregivers. This skill-sharing will increase access to music therapy best practices for those who provide everyday care to people with dementia and other physical and mental health challenges.

- More senior care institutions are developing music therapy services, under the supervision or with the consultation of music therapists, as part of healthcare delivery. This will increase access to music therapy for people with dementia, depression, and other neurological disorders that are well represented in senior care communities.

The Institute for Music and Neurologic Function provides music therapy at a full-service senior care community (Wartburg). In addition, the IMNF serves as a consultant to senior care communities and hospitals that want to use music therapeutically:

- as part of clinical treatment, generally

- in mental health/wellness programming

- in everyday care for people with dementia, and others.

Sometimes, an organization's goal is to develop a music therapy program—beginning with the hiring of a board-certified music therapist. More often, the first step is for the IMNF to share music therapy best practices with recreation therapists, CNAs, HHAs, family care partners, and others, through targeted training.

We can report that, with strong commitment and effective training, a healthcare facility can begin using music therapy best practices throughout the organization, even if it does not have the resources to establish a formal music therapy program.

In this module, we will address an important question: *How can your organization incorporate music therapy best practices in clinical practice and everyday care?* That is, how can you use music therapeutically to improve the healthcare services you provide to patients; to improve the health and wellness of patients; and to realize positive outcomes for your organization—and for yourself?

What do you need in order to get started?

## Setting the stage for success
### Executive leadership—and "champions"
The key to incorporating music therapy best practices in your organization is executive leadership and commitment. Here's why.

Medicare and Medicaid are the primary funders of senior care in the United States, and neither program regularly reimburses senior care institutions for music therapy, except as part of hospice care or the mental health partial hospitalization program. Otherwise, claims are paid on a case-by-case basis, and only if music therapy is deemed medically necessary to reach a treatment goal of an individual patient. It's difficult to prove that music therapy is "medically necessary," though it may indeed be the most effective and least expensive way to achieve a treatment goal in a great many individual cases. In other words, funding music therapy is a challenge. It follows that a healthcare organization serving seniors is unlikely to develop a music therapy program unless its president/CEO or senior leadership has formed a commitment to music therapy based on their values and experience, and on the compelling evidence for music therapy.

The president/CEO is in a position to articulate how music therapy—or staff training in music therapy best practices—will support the organization's mission and core values. The president/CEO must be able to build support from key constituencies within the organization, and from patients and community as well.

Other potential advocates for music therapy initiatives may be board members, and members of the senior leadership team.

### How does support for music therapy happen?
David Gentner, President and CEO of Wartburg, has written: "People working in senior care and service environment know, intuitively and anecdotally, the power of music...as it is generally offered as part of a therapeutic environment in nursing homes, assisted living facilities, and adult day care centers" (Gentner, 2017, p.15).

But as Gentner and others realize, it's not enough to have experienced the power of music intuitively and through interactions with individual patients. The critical next step is to consider the evidence in support of a proposed program: *What does music therapy research tell us about the measurable benefits to specific patient populations? What does experience tell us about the likely benefits to the organization as a whole?*

The value of a music therapy approach will be reflected not only in patient outcomes, but also in the well-being of the organization (including "the bottom line"). Music therapy best practices must be shown to be not only effective, but cost effective. An approach that recognizes all factors has the best chance of enlisting other potential advocates for music therapy, including board members, administrators, and clinical leaders.

## A closer look

Currently, music therapy is offered (sometimes as "integrative" or "complementary" medicine) through various clinical services at top-rated US hospitals like Johns Hopkins Hospital (which has a Center for Music and Medicine), NYU-Langone Hospitals, the Cleveland Clinic, Mayo Clinic, Mount Sinai Beth Israel of New York (which hosts the innovative Louis Armstrong Department of Music Therapy), and Houston Methodist Hospital (which has established the Center for Performing Arts Medicine as part of its Environment of Care program), among others. Music therapy is becoming part of mainstream medicine—if a small part, for now.

It's not surprising that many presidents/CEOs of senior care organizations, too, are exploring music therapy (and other creative arts therapies). Gentner is an example: his academic work includes a dissertation on "Music and Dementia: A Caregiver's Perspective of the Effects of Individualized Music Programming on Quality of Life for Seniors Living in Assisted Living Environments" (Gentner, 2017). In this study, Gentner was able to measure and interpret the results of an important music intervention, with reference to clinical research and his own experience. As a researcher, he recognized the limitations of music therapy research—the need for more studies and with larger subject populations. But as President/CEO, he also understood how best to apply the emerging evidence in the real environment of a nursing home or assisted living facility.

The presidents/CEOs of healthcare organizations are necessarily well versed in the business side of operations, and often in health policy as well. Today, they are increasingly aware of the role of "the science of arts, health, and well-being," as it is sometimes called. And they may be ready to become champions of music therapy.

## Other "champions"

Music therapy best practices also need "champions" within your healthcare organization, and in the community. You can identify and reach out to these champions, solicit their ideas, and enlist their support.

A champion might be a staff neurologist or physician who has discovered that music can help her communicate with patients; a speech and language pathologist who was elated by the progress of the few patients who were offered music therapy; a recreation therapist and army veteran who observed the therapeutic power of music in a combat environment... Champions are there, within your organization. You only need to find them.

And there may be champions in the community as well: people who, based on their own lived experience, are primed to support a music therapy program in a healthcare facility that serves the community.

## A community leader takes action: Judy's story

For community leader Judy Simon, music therapy was a no-brainer. With more than 25 years of experience in the health care industry, she had seen first-hand how music positively affected different populations.

Working with patients with Alzheimer's disease, Judy had watched their responses as musicians were playing the piano or singing familiar songs. She observed that patients' anxiety levels diminished and their mood improved. She noticed, too, that the music triggered memories within many of the patients, and that they began to communicate better.

The more she watched, the more Judy began to believe in the healing power of music. She was convinced that music therapy would be a natural addition to a hospital setting.

Judy became committed to bringing a music therapy program to her community hospital, Northern Westchester Hospital (NWH), a highly rated not-for-profit hospital, located in Mount Kisco, NY, about 45 miles north of New York City.

### Turning a vision into a reality

After meeting with the hospital, Judy understood the importance of having a credible, evidence-based music therapy program that would work with hospital clinicians to create a truly unique and outcomes-based program. Input from a music therapist was essential. The Institute for Music and Neurology Function, an internationally renowned center of music therapy treatment, research, and education, was located in the Bronx, not too far away. Following up on Judy's recommendation, the hospital initiated a partnership with the IMNF to design a program that met their institutional needs.

Among those who participated in the planning team were the chief executive officer, chief operations officer, senior administrators, and department heads.

The planning process was an education for everyone.

The more the team learned about individuals who were helped by music therapy, the more convinced they were that music therapy would enhance the quality of life for patients and visitors at NWH. Later, hospital staff would share with Judy that they didn't really appreciate the power of music until they saw it in action with patients. A staff member described how a patient who had been very lethargic opened his eyes and started interacting when he heard his favorite rock and roll song being played, and how a very depressed patient who had come from a nursing home actively engaged and became full of life when a childhood lullaby was played.

As one nurse stated, "The renewed energy that patients feel after the music therapy experience creates a sense of empowerment and willingness to take control of their recovery."

Judy's passion transformed her into a woman on a mission. To help cover the program expenses, she began knocking on doors, soliciting donations, and gaining support for a concept that she believed would make a difference in the lives of patients and families at NWH. In 2010, Judy Simon's vision became a reality when the music therapy program was launched at Northern Westchester Hospital. In 2011, the Music Therapy program at NWH received the 2011 National Spirit of Planetree Award for Best Practice Program, for its support of the hospital's mission of improving the health and wellness of its community members through the power of song. (And that was just the beginning... (Adapted from the in-house publication "Music Therapy: The Healing Power of Music. Developing a Hospital Music Therapy Program," Northern Westchester Hospital, Mount Kisco, New York, 2012)

## TAKEAWAYS

Judy Simon was clearly an extraordinary community leader. Yet the story of Northern Westchester Hospital has relevance for other healthcare facilities at a time when community interest around healthcare is at an all-time high.

Are there champions for music therapy, and music and arts programming, in your community? Are they connected to your organization—as board members, staff, volunteers, or patient families? As past donors or likely supporters? (Volunteers like Judy Simon tend to move easily into leadership once committed to a cause.) If you can identify potential champions, the next step is to reach out and have a conversation about how a music therapy program would improve the health and wellness of the community. Of course, this requires at least one champion to initiate the effort. *Is that you?*

To make her vision a reality, Simon consulted early on with experienced music therapists at the Institute of Music and Neurologic Function. As a rule, a healthcare organization that is planning a music therapy program, even a small program, should consult with a certified music therapist to ensure that the proposed program is evidence-based, responsive to clinical needs, and respectful of available resources.

## A commitment to person-centered care

**A music therapy program is most likely to thrive in a senior care community that is committed to "person-centered care."** This is an approach to care that is based on treating every person in care with empathy, sensitivity, and acceptance (Clemons, 2021). **In person-centered care, quality of life is a core value; and what constitutes quality of life is understood to be unique to each person.** Care must therefore be personalized to allow for individual choices, and as much independence (autonomy) as possible, for patients in short- or long-term care, and at every level of functioning.

Person-centered care extends to patients' family and care partners, who are welcomed into the care setting. And it's an approach that, in the best instances, characterizes the whole organization. A person-centered healthcare system recognizes that staff, as well as patients, experience higher quality of life when able to express choices and maintain meaningful control of the nature, timing, and pace of their daily activities.

If you work in senior care, you've probably heard a lot about person-centered (or patient-centered) care. These are standard models of care that are expected to be the norm in residential facilities.

In practice, meeting the high standards of person-centered care presents challenges to staff at all levels. The main challenge, as any caregiver will tell you, is finding the time to listen and pay full attention to each person's needs; the time to establish the communication that underlies a trusting relationship. And then there is the challenge of actually responding to that person's needs, with flexible care schedules, food choices, and the like. Not easy. Yet, when we institute music therapy best practices, it's not long before we see CNAs taking time to sing to their patients, as they go about daily care activities. What is going on there?

Music therapy works to support the person-centered care model. And vice versa: When person-centered care is well implemented in a senior care setting, music therapy best practices can be part of that success. Here's why:

- **Music therapy is a personalized (or "individualized") approach, providing not just music, but the right music for a specific person, at a time (and in a manner) that is right for that person.** For example: personalized playlists figure importantly in music interventions for seniors in care. These playlists are just that: "personalized" or "person-centered." They reflect the person's life experience, family, and cultural background. You have to know and interview a person, or a family member, to put together a playlist that has the potential to be therapeutic for your patient. When you do that, you are taking a person-centered approach to the person in your care. We suggest that there is nothing you will hand to your patient, in the course of daily care, that is as personal as the iPad that delivers your patient's personal music.

- **Music therapy best practices greatly expand the possibilities for communication between patients and caregivers, which is a foundation of person-centered care.** In a long-term care community, an important role of the music therapist is to train CNAs, HHAs, and family care partners to use familiar songs and music to reach people living with dementia and other neurological conditions. As is well established, music, as a nonverbal language, often gets through when words alone do not (see Module 6 for examples of music interventions in daily care). Because music has rich autobiographical associations for most people, music interventions delivered in group sessions are effective in addressing symptoms of depression and other common mental health issues among seniors in care. These interventions, out of clinical necessity, are always *personalized* or *person-centered*.

- **Senior care facilities that sign on to person-centered care do not favor interventions that medicate or restrain patients to ensure compliance with care regimes—not if other options are available. Research suggests that person-centered ("individualized") music programming is a non-pharmacological intervention that has the potential to improve the quality of life for people living with dementia, including those with moderate to severe dementia, who represent a significant population in assisted living and residential care** (Gentner, 2017).

In particular, music therapy has proven to be effective in preventing some of the behavioral and psychological symptoms of dementia (most notably, anxiety). You can understand why this is important; it has been said that, even for caregivers who are on board with person-centered values, the overarching goal is often to have a calm resident in a controlled environment (Kolanowski *et al.*, 2010, cited in Gentner, 2017, p.22). Music interventions that defuse anxiety and prevent aggression are welcomed by caregivers, who may be dealing with their own anxieties. The music, shared within a relationship, has the potential to relieve anxiety in both patient and caregiver. In a range of everyday experiences, rhythmic music and singing have been shown to bring patient and caregiver in sync with each other—as is reported by caregivers themselves.

The experience of the IMNF, over 20 years, with diverse residential and adult day-care programs, suggests that music interventions may reduce the need for anti-depressants and pain medications among patients. Clinical research in the field supports these observations, in ways that increasingly shape clinical care.

## A music-rich environment

It's easiest to introduce therapeutic music programs in a senior care facility that already has a music-rich environment. That's partly because the staff will have had opportunities to observe the positive effects of music on patients in recreational contexts: so there is likely to be strong staff buy-in for anything that brings "more music." Live performances by visiting musicians and community groups, community singalongs, and outings to local concerts, musical theatre, and opera are always popular in senior settings, and can be observed to raise mood and morale among residents at all levels of function (and among staff as well). An institution that highlights these activities is signaling the high value it places on music, as part of the therapeutic environment.

A music-rich environment is also likely to have in place the resources to support music therapy best practices. Among the necessary resources are musical instruments, audio equipment, technical support for music activities, and volunteer support from amateur and professional musicians, community music groups, teaching artists, and others.

A music-rich environment is where we are most likely to see a physical therapist or transportation aide pushing a patient in a wheelchair, while singing along the way, or a patient with dementia who is singing in the day room, along with a musician volunteer who has found a song for her.

## ABOUT YOU

### Are you working in a music-rich senior care environment?

How many of the music activities listed below have you observed or participated in over the past three months? Check *Yes* for activities that you have observed or participated in at least once, and *double check* those activities that are regularly offered in your work environment.

### Recreational music, and entertainment:

- Live performances by professional or amateur musical group for residents in common spaces
  Yes_____

- Live performances by musicians in day rooms or on residential floors
  Yes_____

- Arranged visits for residents or patients to community music events (concerts, musical theatre, opera)
  Yes_____

### Music activities and community events that have the potential:

- Recorded music offered as a background for pleasurable dining
  Yes_____

- Recorded music offered in waiting rooms and other clinical areas
  Yes_____

### Recreation therapy programming that prioritizes music-accompanied exercises and activities, including:

- Singalongs or choirs for residents in general
  Yes_____

- Singalongs or choirs for people with dementia and their caregivers or family care partners
  Yes_____

- Drumming circles (or therapeutic drumming circles) for community in general
  Yes_____

- Drumming circles (or therapeutic drumming circles) for people with dementia and their caregivers or for family care partners
  Yes_____

- A personalized playlist program for people with dementia, and others
  Yes_____

## TAKEAWAY

What have you learned about the role of music in your work environment?

- How many of the music activities listed are regularly provided?

- What, if any, effects do they have on you (your mood, your relationships with patients, your ability to do your job, etc.)?

- If you have worked in other senior care settings, how would you compare the level of music activity in your current work environment with what you have experienced elsewhere?

## A creative aging approach

Music therapy best practices thrive in an environment that offers a range of arts-based programs as part of "creative aging" and lifetime learning. In such an environment, arts activities are not primarily recreational; they are opportunities for learning and personal development. We are used to viewing music, dance, and art lessons as valuable experiences for children and young people—and so they are for older people, too.

Creative aging programs provide quality arts education and arts experiences, taught by professionals, or "teaching artists." Participants build art-making skills over time; the experience can be life changing, helping older people, including those in residential and adult day programs, to remain challenged and engaged in life. Reported benefits include greater social engagement, increased self-esteem, and a sense of accomplishment, and often joy, in art-making.

A creative aging model that has received awards and international recognition is Wartburg's Creative Aging and Lifetime Learning Initiative. Founded in 2011, the program offers high-quality, multi-week programs in a variety of disciplines. Current offerings include drawing and painting, ceramics, quilting, choral singing, African drumming, technology class, oral and video history, and more. As to music and dance, Wartburg has taken creative aging to a new level. These programs are led by music and dance therapists. This allows Wartburg to offer *arts-based programs with a therapeutic design*.

Music therapists and dance therapists are creative arts therapists, a recognized category of health professionals who are certified to use a specific art form in therapeutic practice. Music therapy is the most established of the creative arts therapies. Among the arts, music has been most fully studied with respect to its effects on health and wellness. Clinical experience in music therapy extends over 75 years; and recent research on music and the brain is providing new insights into the (potential) effectiveness of music therapy in the treatment of neurological diseases.

**Adding a music therapist to an arts-based program at the creative aging level can be a first step toward establishing a music therapy program in a senior care setting.** The addition of a music therapist (and other creative arts therapists) creates an art-based program with a therapeutic design; that in turn means that art-making experiences can address specific health and wellness issues that are not within the "scope of practice" of professional teaching artists. As an example, a professional dancer and teaching artist can offer participants a stimulating dance session that will have many therapeutic effects—higher energy, better balance, improved mood, an aesthetic experience, and so on. But a music or dance therapist can offer interventions that address falls prevention in frail seniors, and the needs of participants with Parkinson's disease and other movement disorders.

The last five years have seen a growing interest in "advancing the sciences of arts, health and wellness." The World Health Organization established an Arts and Health Program in 2019. And the National Institute on Aging of the NIH has informed us that "Participating in the arts creates paths to healthy aging" (2019). It seems inevitable that arts-based programming in senior care will expand in response to this trending awareness. Music therapy programs can share resources with these programs, as they develop.

## Types of arts and health practices

With so much happening on the arts in healthcare front, it is sometimes difficult to distinguish between the practitioners and programs emerging in this area.

For our purposes, it's useful to focus on two groups of practitioners, as described by the National Organization for Arts in Health:

- Creative arts therapies: This includes the distinct, regulated health professions of art therapy, dance/movement therapy, drama therapy, music therapy, poetry therapy, and psychodrama therapy. These are board-certified fields, with clearly defined standards of practice and educational requirements, each using a specific art form and delivery method as treatment. These fields are rooted in the belief that each form of therapy has limited therapeutic value unless it is administered under precise protocols and conditions.

- Arts in health programs: Located within medical centers and other healthcare institutions, these include visiting artists, artists-in-residence, arts programming developed in partnership with community arts agencies, arts collections, and rotating arts exhibits (National Organization for Arts in Health, 2017). Most creative aging programs would fall into this category.

## A sound-friendly environment

A tenet of person-centered care is that every person should be able to exercise personal choice in the care environment, to the fullest extent possible. In a hospital, a doctor's office, or a long-term care facility, we want to have some control over the environment—how it feels and how we experience it.

People experience the world through the senses. That being so, we recognize that it is important for residents in a senior care facility to have some control over the food they taste, the colors and pictures in their room, the room temperature and lighting, and the sounds in their environment. Of these sensory experiences, sound is famously the least responsive to our control—so much so that we often speak of being "assaulted" by aversive sound or "noise." In a residential facility or hospital, patients typically are subjected to noise levels that cause a significant level of discomfort. Noise may also interfere with communication and social interactions, and have adverse effects on attention, cognition, and much else.

Music is part of the sound environment. Interestingly, an ambitious project funded by the National Institutes of Health is called The Sound Health Initiative, and its overarching goal is to "bring together music therapy and neuroscience" (see Module 1).

In a residential facility, our goal must be to create an environment that supports "sound health" for both residents and staff. That is, we must apply what we know from music therapy and neuroscience research to design a sound environment that supports health and wellness. Music will be part of that environment.

To bring music therapy best practices to your care setting, it is advisable to assess, and, as necessary, improve, the sound environment. What follows are suggestions for creating a sound environment in line with music therapy best practices.

### Television audio

Almost always, it is necessary to rethink television use in common areas. In many residential care facilities, television audio is constant and pervasive. Typically, in the day room, maybe 90 percent of the residents are not attending to the visuals on the screen, as evidenced by lack of eye contact, and they do not appear to be responding to the audio either. The volume may not be loud, but seldom is it modulated to take into account the time of day or concurrent activities. When live music is presented by a visiting musician or musician volunteer, the television audio is a distracting background (of course it should be muted). Unmonitored television audio may cause agitation and irritability in some patients, withdrawal in others.

In a healthy sound environment, music-based TV or videos can be used therapeutically to stimulate cognitive function, social interaction, and movement; to give pleasure and a sense of community. This can happen when staff are trained to use the TV or video experience to engage a specific patient audience. Music therapy best practices focus on using music *intentionally* in the care environment.

## Background noise

To establish a sound environment that welcomes music, it is necessary to reduce extraneous background noises as much as possible. Constant humming from large refrigerators and other equipment, squeaking and rattling of wheels on maintenance carts, and unrelieved kitchen and serving clatter in dining areas require attention. These uncontrolled noises may cause agitation, attention issues, and confusion in some patients, and are to some degree stressful to everyone, including staff. And, of course, they interfere with music activities.

Distracting noises that are a necessary part of daily operations may need to be reviewed. Shrill alarms (often not immediately attended to) might require closer oversight. Over-loud announcements on the public address system should be avoided. Loud conversations and other noises associated with shift changes should be minimized.

If music is played as background in dining areas, staff should observe the effect on residents of the music selected, with guidance from a music therapist, if available, and with reference to music therapy best practices. Familiar music that is not overly stimulating will usually be recommended.

## The *sound* of music

To create a sound environment for music, it is necessary to monitor the sound systems and instruments that are used in music programming for quality purposes. Put simply, *the music must sound good*. The goal is a clear and pleasing tone, and dynamics that can be modulated for expressive purposes. Make sure that pianos are tuned; that speakers are adequate and free of static.

For singalongs, choose a leader who has a pleasant voice and can engage participants in a meaningful way. Leadership skills as well as music skills are important. For performances, seek out community musicians and groups that have been vetted and found to be musically competent and well suited for your acoustical space.

You might ask, why does this matter? Many of your patients may lack experience or current ability to discriminate (consciously) between good or not-so-good music, based on performance values. But music therapy tells us that you don't have to know anything about music, or be functioning at a level that engages your critical abilities, to know what sounds good.

Consider this: almost everyone responds to a "beautiful voice," and to a speaker who uses dynamics and rhythms expressively. The content is often not the point: as history shows, whole populations respond to charismatic leaders and demagogues who have mastered the rhythm, melody, and dynamics of persuasive speech. We do not respond the same way to a speaker or singer who has a flat, toneless voice and an uncertain rhythm. In fact, music of poor quality can be distracting, potentially undermining the beneficial effects of music listening or participation.

## TAKEAWAY
Good sound quality, and high music values, are important to all music listeners, including people with dementia and other cognitive or education deficits.

### Other environmental concerns
To support music-based activities, a healthcare facility needs adequate, easily accessible storage facilities for musical instruments and equipment. Special care must be taken to ensure that instruments are safely stored, and maintained as needed. Choose storage spaces that are not subject to high humidity, dryness, or drastic changes in temperature or humidity.

A growing music program will also require abundant and accessible charging stations for technical devices, and carts to support mobility of instruments and equipment to floor units.

## Moving it forward: Implementing your plan
### Building commitment and institutional buy-in
### for music therapy best practices
When the president/CEO and senior leadership make a commitment to incorporate music therapy best practices in senior care, the next step is to build commitment throughout the organization. Everyone's mission is to

improve the quality of care. So you will need "institutional buy-in" from staff at all levels for an innovation that will affect patient care as well as some management practices.

Music therapy "champions," including music therapists involved in the project, will need to build interest and support from these key groups:

- Heads of all departments who will need to sign off on the implementation of music therapy best practices affecting their patients, especially supervisors of staff members who will deliver music interventions, as part of patient care (for example, director of nursing, director of rehabilitation).

- Frontline caregivers who will deliver music interventions (recreation therapists, CNAs, HHAs).

- Members of the healthcare team who will collaborate in the delivery of music interventions. (This may include recreational therapists, physical therapists, occupational therapists, speech and language pathologists, social workers, etc., depending on the patient population to be served.)

It is also important to engage management staff who will be affected by the innovation, including human resources officers, who will be involved in staff hiring and staff satisfaction issues, and maintenance staff and technicians, who will be charged with maintaining spaces and equipment for expanded music activities.

## Making the case: The importance of first-hand experience

The best way to make the case for music therapy best practices in your senior care organization is to offer a music intervention to staff (especially caregiving staff). Participation in a music intervention makes the most direct and convincing case for the therapeutic power of music; experiencing the music intervention first hand will motivate staff to learn more about music therapy best practices, and apply them to patient care.

- Frontline caregivers might participate in a therapeutic drumming circle, a rhythmic activity, or a wellness group led by music therapists, as part of an introduction to music interventions. The music therapist, as group leader, will model best practices, and perhaps follow with a discussion or debriefing.

- If the organization already offers a personalized playlist program for dementia patients, caregiving staff may draw on their experience with this intervention to more broadly support music therapy best practices in senior care. For the general public, there has been no more powerful argument for music in senior care than the videos and first-hand reports about people with dementia who "come alive" after months or years of silence and immobility, on hearing a piece of favorite music. To generate interest in music therapy best practices, you may want to circulate relevant videos, and stories and memoirs of caregivers.

## Partnering with therapeutic recreation

Gaining support from therapeutic recreation is a priority. And usually it's a win-win. When it comes to music-based activities, recreation therapists are the most knowledgeable members of the healthcare team—and the first to express interest in learning new music skills. Many (but not all) recreation therapists play the guitar or keyboard, and all use recorded music in recreation programming. In other words, they've had first-hand experience. "There is no problem in convincing people in recreation therapy as to the benefits of music," says a chief of recreation therapy at a major Veterans Affairs hospital. "You see it all the time." Music *is* "a big piece" of recreation therapy, he adds, especially now with iPods and Alexa ready to deliver recorded music (Bonadies, V., personal communication, May 9, 2022).

Recreation therapists are likely to support the implementation of music therapy best practices, providing their concerns are addressed. The main concern is finding the time to implement new music-based activities, often in the face of staff shortages.

It should be possible to demonstrate that implementing music therapy best practices will provide *additional resources* to recreation therapists who are involved in delivering music activities. The music therapist who is engaged as a consultant or staff member will introduce intentional music activities to build on therapeutic recreation programming, and in most cases will train additional staff (CNAs) to deliver music activities.

## Gaining support from clinical leaders and caregiving staff

To enlist the support of clinical leaders, you might begin by increasing awareness about "the project"—what it will mean to institute music therapy best practices in patient care in your organization. In cases where this involves establishing a music therapy program or department, it will be easy to announce and call attention to this effort. In other cases, it is helpful if the project has a title that is appropriate to organizational goals. For example, "Music Therapy Best Practices for Dementia Care" or "Music for Senior Health and Wellness."

Here are some ways to generate enthusiasm and support:

- In preparation for the project launch, reach out to educate staff about the benefits of music therapy innovations for patients, staff, and the organization as a whole.

  - Circulate articles, and links to online stories and videos, that make a strong case for music therapy best practices in settings similar to yours. Curate your outreach, with content that is brief, relevant, and stimulating. If possible, provide a means for staff to respond and follow up on all responses.

  - **Show how the project will support the core values and mission of the organization, and how it will interface with other initiatives that have improved patient outcomes, and patient satisfaction.** (For example, does the project build on a successful creative aging program?) Interviews with clinical leaders, patients, and patient advocates are a possibility.

- Reach out to medical and nursing leaders with research articles on the latest evidence regarding music interventions in their practice areas. Ask for responses; create a dialogue between disciplines.

- When the project is underway, invite targeted staff members to observe music therapy best practices in action, in a music-based group or intervention. Help them see and understand the impact on the patients who participate.

- As the project develops, share success stories—informative, inspiring stories that personalize the therapeutic work—in your organization's newsletters, on the website, and through emails and flyers. Building awareness is an ongoing process.

### Welcoming CNAs and HHAs as partners

As noted, first-hand experience makes the best case for music interventions. And this is especially true for frontline caregivers. **It may be difficult for CNAs and HHAs to anticipate the benefits of using music therapy best practices (*when they have so much else to do!*). But many caregivers, once they have participated in training and have had some experience on the floor, are enthusiastic about using music in patient care.**

Research on caregiver satisfaction with music-based care has focused mainly on caregivers of patients with moderate to severe dementia and others who need help with activities of daily living. In the US, these caregivers are mostly CNAs who work in long-term care. (Much of the research in this area has been conducted in the UK, Canada, and Sweden, nations that are ahead of the US in instituting music-based care programs.) A few studies and much anecdotal evidence have come from family care partners as well.

The research shows that using music therapy best practices reduces what is too often called "the burden of caregiving." Caregivers, as well as patients, benefit from music interventions. They report that music makes it easier to communicate with patients, defuse problems, and complete the day's activities together. Caregiver singing, and rhythmic humming and movement, help the CNA and the person with dementia move together, in tune and in time with each other. The person with dementia becomes more engaged, more "present," and the caregiver feels empowered.

Training in music therapy best practices teaches caregivers how to blend rhythmic activities into everyday acts of care—to "Sing while you comb hair, play music during bathing time. Hum when putting the resident to bed for the evening" (Institute for Music and Neurologic Function, 2007). In this caregiving scenario, there is less confusion, less resistance to care on the part of the person with dementia, and, significantly, there is less agitation (see Module 6).

## Among the outcomes
### Less agitation experienced by patients

Best practices in music therapy for senior care are evidence-based; and **there is strong evidence that caregiver-initiated music is effective in reducing agitation in people with moderate to severe dementia. Other music interventions, such as the use of personal playlists or engagement around familiar songs, have also been shown to be effective in reducing agitation, and other behaviors that originate in anxiety and fear.** What caregiver would not welcome a tool that helped them reduce patient anxiety, and the chances of verbal or physical aggression in the care situation? Indeed, the support for funding for music therapy has tended to focus on its effectiveness in treating behavioral and psychological symptoms of dementia.

### Reduced use of antipsychotic medications

Much of the research on the effectiveness of music interventions is based on caregivers' reports. But we can also look to the clinical record, with the goal of measuring the effects or outcomes of music interventions.

One interesting measure is the use of antipsychotic medications, a class of medications developed to treat serious mental illnesses that are commonly used (and misused) to reduce anxiety in people with dementia. The evidence shows that music therapy, as delivered through various music interventions, reduces the need for antipsychotic medications for people with dementia, and for other nursing home residents. For example, in the UK, a major study of music-based interventions for people with dementia found that music therapy reduced the need for antipsychotic medication in 67 percent of people with dementia (Meadows & McLennan, 2022).

You may be able to identify similar outcomes in your own organization. At Wartburg, which supports a creative aging program as well as music therapy, the use of antipsychotic drugs is well below state and national levels.

Music interventions, including personalized playlists, elicit memories, personal responses, and often social interactions—*without almost no side effects*. In a music interaction, the nursing home resident is typically engaged and "present," which results in easier, more rewarding caregiving. By contrast, antipsychotic medications often blunt personality, impair communication, and have other negative effects on a person's relationships with caregivers and others. (And these medications potentially have harmful physical side effects as well.)

### Benefits for caregivers

The research, *much of it based on reports of caregivers*, will be of interest to CNAs and HHAs in your organization. In a person-centered care environment, caregiving staff are receptive to acquiring new skills that will promote better patient care; and they will contribute ideas and recommendations, based on their experience. A training program in music therapy best practices is potentially a growth experience for participants—it will likely enhance their performance, confidence, and self-esteem in the care environment, and possibly in other areas of life as well. The healthcare team will benefit, in turn, from what caregivers tell them about their experience.

The truth is that music is potentially therapeutic for caregivers as well as patients. As one caregiver puts it, the music is not just for the resident: "It lifts your mood as well" (Bowell & Bamford, 2018, p.39).

Sometimes, a music intervention promotes staff wellness and feelings of community throughout the facility. See, for example, participants' evaluation of therapeutic drumming and rhythm activities. (See Module 2: "It's the number one interdisciplinary team vitamin.")

It's not surprising that during the Covid-19 pandemic, some hospitals offered therapeutic music groups to staff to reduce stress and promote wellness and self-care. Given the high staff turnover in nursing homes and other facilities, even in ordinary times, this is an idea well worth considering.

### Cost-effectiveness: Can we make the case?

The evidence base for music therapy and music therapy best practices has grown impressively in recent years. Much of the research has focused on the healthcare needs of those who are the largest consumers of healthcare services—people 65 and over. Older people account for the greatest expenditure of healthcare dollars by the US government. And yet in music therapy, *as in other areas of healthcare*, our research (cutting edge as it may be) falls short when it comes to addressing cost-effectiveness issues.

We expend our resources on determining what is effective in treating various conditions. And sometimes, even if we don't yet have strong evidence, we are willing to take large (and costly) chances on medical interventions *if there are people in need of help and advocates for helping them through a therapy at hand,* and if the risk seems manageable. Surgery for back pain (does it work?); stents for heart disease (do they reduce the risks for patients who are not experiencing an emergency?); multiple anti-depressants for adolescent depression (is there a better way?). We are willing to support interventions when there is some good evidence ("a chance") that they may relieve suffering, extend life, and promote well-being for the people we love. For these costly interventions, we require only the evidence we think we need; and we don't say much about cost effectiveness.

What we don't seem able to do is support "non-medical" interventions, like music therapy, on these same grounds. Music therapy—like surgical and pharmacological interventions—has been shown to relieve suffering, extend life, and promote well-being (or quality of life). The call for more studies is justified, to be sure, and more studies are underway. But in the meantime should we not be willing to take a chance on music therapy, *if there are people in need of help, and good evidence that music therapy will help them, at little or no risk?* If the answer is yes, or maybe, do we need to look at costs, even as we recognize that medical, surgical, and pharmacological interventions are not always under the same scrutiny? *Of course we do.*

## Here is what we know about the cost-effectiveness of music therapy

We can say with authority that music therapy, as a treatment modality in senior care, is relatively inexpensive. At the high end, the cost of employing a full-time music therapist as a staff member in senior care is about $95,000 a year, or the equivalent of $46.00 an hour—roughly the same as for an occupational therapist. In skilled nursing facilities, salaries of staff music therapists will align more closely with recreation therapists, which is about $60,000 a year, and often lower. We should note that in senior care facilities, many music therapists work part time or on a per diem basis; the hourly fee for part-time work is about $70–100 an hour, for both group and individual sessions. Training CNAs and other staff to use music therapy best practices results in costs that are lower still. The IMNF's experience shows that a music therapy program can be launched and developed with a single, experienced music therapist and a well-grounded training program.

**Music interventions, delivered by music therapists or trained staff, are both inexpensive and easy to administer. And there is little risk involved.** Music therapy potentially has many positive effects (as demonstrated by research and clinical experience), and almost no harmful (or costly) side effects (see Module 1). Never does music therapy result in the need for costly additional treatment or hospitalization (as some invasive procedures or medications do).

From a business perspective, we might also note that music engagement, as achieved through music therapy best practices, is a positive experience for most patients; as such it contributes to patient and family satisfaction, and to a facility's efforts to connect to the community. Our experience at the IMNF has shown that the message that "Music is everywhere" can be effective in marketing a care facility to families in the communities served.

The research on the cost-effectiveness of music therapy is not extensive, partly because there are few sources of funding for such research. Still, it is possible to suggest areas in which music therapy best practices have been shown to be good for the bottom line.

Below are some findings that may be of interest to senior care organizations that are ready to institute music therapy best practices.

- As noted, music interventions have been shown to reduce the need for antipsychotic medications for people living with dementia and for other nursing home residents. We might ask, does the use of music, as opposed to medication, also result in cost savings, and to what extent? The NeuroArts Blueprint, an initiative that seeks to broadly advance "the science of arts, health and wellbeing," was interested in this question. It engaged KPMG, an international professional services and accounting organization, to prepare an economic analysis of musical engagement as a strategy to ease the symptoms of Alzheimer's disease (KPMG, 2021).

  In this study, music engagement included any type of music session (e.g. singing, listening to music, playing a musical instrument, etc.) occurring in an individual or group setting, with the intention of improving the health and well-being of people living with Alzheimer's disease. **KPMG found that music engagement costs are "far less costly" compared to pharmacological treatments for [symptoms of] Alzheimer's disease.**

  From study assumptions, annual music engagement costs in 2020 were about $802 per person with Alzheimer's disease, regardless of disease severity, as opposed to annual per-person prescription costs of approximately $3500 (as estimated by the Alzheimer's Association).

In other words, music engagement costs less than a quarter of what might (otherwise) be spent on medication.

The study also highlighted broad economic benefits derived from the assumptions. For example, it is suggested that with a 50 percent adoption rate, participation of people with Alzheimer's disease in music engagement could contribute a total of $1.4 billion to GDP. Another interesting effect would be the increased employee income that would be earned by unpaid caregivers (family care partners) who are able to work more paid hours due to improvements in the health and well-being of people with Alzheimer's. *What does that tell us?*

This study is the first to look at the economic benefits of music engagement for people living with Alzheimer's disease in the US. Further study is needed. It is significant that other nations that have studied the matter in the context of their own healthcare systems are moving to fold funding for music therapy into customary senior care. In Australia, music therapy is included in various State and Commonwealth Government programs, including state-funded hospitals and mental health services. An official recommendation required that "residential aged care...employ or otherwise retain" at least one music or art therapist by June 2024.

- Evidence for the cost-effectiveness of music therapy in senior care has come from the PACE program (the Program of All-Inclusive Care for the Elderly). PACE serves older people who are eligible for nursing home care but are able to live at home with PACE support. Patients served by PACE are living with dementia, mobility problems, chronic diseases, and the health consequences of social isolation. Music therapy (provided by music therapists) has been found to be a cost-effective therapy for these patients. That's not surprising (to us). Because of the way that PACE is funded, the PACE experience with music therapy sends a message to senior care providers.

PACE is a capitated program; it reimburses the provider a set amount for each patient. Since the amount will not increase, there is a powerful motive to prevent adverse events, such as falls or non-compliance with medical regimens (which might lead to costly hospitalization, loss of function, and much suffering). To be successful (financially) as a program model, PACE must optimize health while reducing expenses. Of course, that is true for most healthcare providers. But there's a difference: the PACE program, as established by the Centers for Medicare and Medicaid, has wide latitude in choosing how to spend funds. (If the PACE healthcare team decides that a person needs care and services that Medicare and Medicaid don't cover, PACE may still cover these services.)

In this model, it makes sense for PACE administrators to choose music therapy as a treatment modality. The IMNF's experience with one of the nation's leading PACE programs shows that music therapy is a *low-cost, highly effective way* of reducing the healthcare costs associated with social isolation and depression symptoms; and with the behavioral and psychological symptoms experienced by people with some level of dementia. In addition, music therapy reduces the caregiver burden for PACE staff as well as home-based caregivers. The same benefits are observed in medical day-care programs and in hospice care (in which music therapy is often included as part of the Medicare hospice care plan).

- There is growing recognition in the field of music therapy and critical care medicine that personalized music (i.e. live or recorded music selected by patients) has positive effects on patients undergoing and recovering from surgery. In a 2015 study, published in the prestigious English medical journal *The Lancet*, researchers cited more than 70 well-designed studies that showed that the use of patient-selected recorded music for patients undergoing surgery resulted in a decrease in the need for sedatives and opiate pain relievers (Hole *et al.*, 2015).

In the US, we are seeing research reports, as well as personal memoirs, about the therapeutic and seemingly life-saving effects of music for people who are struggling to emerge from critical care situations. This research is not directly relevant to most senior care facilities. But it is worth noting that in critical care, as in other settings that haven't been as well studied, music that is selected by (or for) the patient has the potential to reduce pain, reduce the need for sedatives and opiate pain relievers, and promote recovery, with potential savings of healthcare dollars across the system.

## The cost benefits that remain invisible

Music therapy-informed groups that focus on social isolation, emotional issues, and depression symptoms are relatively inexpensive. As "non-medical" services, they are perceived as "extras," and not generally reimbursable by Medicare or Medicaid. But these groups are very effective in addressing major health problems.

As we will see (Module 4), social isolation has profound consequences for physical and mental health, not just for older people, but for all of us.

With reference to older people, a comprehensive review of the research finds that a "particularly devastating" consequence of feeling socially isolated is cognitive decline and dementia (Hawkley & Cacioppo, 2010). Loneliness is also associated with increased risk of stroke and coronary heart disease, and with underlying conditions such as high blood pressure and obesity.

In short-term rehabilitation units, we often see people who feel socially isolated and depressed in the aftermath of a stroke, or with the progression of Parkinson's disease, for example. These individuals are often unable to participate in their own rehabilitation due to underlying depression that seems secondary, and goes untreated. We see patients injured in falls, who present with mild cognitive loss, and are unable to fully engage in rehabilitation.

We can provide these patients with a relatively inexpensive music-based therapy group, which will reduce isolation and depression symptoms, support their efforts at recovery, and make it possible for them to return home. If we don't, the next step for these patients may be a nursing home, where they will receive daily care at considerable cost to the system.

So why not music therapy? If you are a senior healthcare administrator, looking at this through a cost-benefit lens, you might notice that the benefit in this case would be realized by the insurance company (or Medicare/Medicaid) which would not have to pay for long-term care. But the healthcare facility that provided the cost-saving intervention—your facility—might also benefit, in becoming a preferred provider of subacute rehab for the insurance providers, and (more importantly) for your community.

## TAKEAWAY

Music therapy, and interventions that reflect music therapy best practices, are cost effective in part because they reduce the effects of depression and social isolation, which contribute very significantly to poor health outcomes among older people, and thus to healthcare costs. The cost savings achieved through music therapy practices are largely invisible—but we must keep them in mind.

## Engaging a music therapist as a consultant, trainer, or member of the healthcare team

Your success in bringing music therapy best practices to your patients or loved one will depend, in large part, on the choice of a music therapist for consultation, training, or hands-on care.

Music therapists may be engaged in several ways, depending on the resources and goals of an organization, an individual, or family. Here are three common models.

- **The music therapist is a consultant or trainer.** Some organizations choose to work with an experienced music therapist or music therapy practice group, as consultants, to plan music-therapy-based programming and train members of the healthcare team in best practices. A music therapy consultant may also help recruit a staff music therapist, if that is part of the plan.

- **The music therapist is a regular staff member, either full or part time.** In this model, the music therapist provides music therapy to patients in a target population, and shares music therapy best practices with other members of the healthcare team. Few senior care facilities have a music therapy service or department, so in most cases the music therapist is part of the therapeutic recreation department or a creative aging program.

  In a variation of this model for private care, a music therapist provides music therapy to a patient at the patient's home, at a professional office, or perhaps virtually. In this model, the music therapist shares their skills with the family care partner. (Note that for families who cannot afford or locate private care, an option is a home health aide who has been trained in music therapy best practices.)

- **The music therapist is a gig worker or freelance** (though sometimes referred to as a "consultant"). In this model, a music therapist might come to a senior care site several times a week to conduct a program or group. Skill-sharing or collaboration with the healthcare team is likely to be minimal.


## Choosing a music therapist consultant or consultant group

As you initiate music therapy best practices at your facility, there are two points at which to engage a music therapist: early in the planning process, to work with the organization's senior leadership and board in designing the project; or at the implementation stage, as you train staff in music therapy best practices and begin to deliver services.

Some organizations choose to work with an experienced music therapist or music therapy practice group, as consultants, during the planning process. In some cases, a consultant will go on to implement music therapy best practices as a staff member. In other cases, the consultant will help recruit (and possibly supervise) the music therapist, who will implement best practices.

If no consultant has been engaged, the organization will recruit a music therapist directly, for a full- or part-time position.

## Qualifications of a music therapist

**It is critical to engage a board-certified music therapist to deliver music therapy or training in music therapy best practices. Certification is denoted by the initials "MT-BC" after the person's name.**

Music therapists with the MT-BC credential have completed a total of 1200 hours of in-depth supervised *clinical training*, including internships in healthcare and education facilities, and have passed a board exam. Every one of these candidates will have advanced music skills, in accompaniment, improvisation, composition, and performance. Music therapists may also receive advanced training in master's or doctoral programs.

*Is it critical to hire a music therapist who has specialized senior care?* We don't think so. All certified music therapists are trained to provide therapy to senior populations, including patients in dementia care and rehabilitation. Music therapy training takes into account a developmental reality—which is that people at all stages of life respond to the same music interventions, adapted and personalized for them as music therapists are trained to do. Even so, many music therapists seek out additional training in order to meet the special needs of people in long-term care facilities. The IMNF has offered advanced training (for credit), and is creating a training program for music therapists who seek advanced certification in areas of long-term care.

Recruitment of a music therapist can begin in your community, as you reach out to local colleges and music schools. To locate nearby schools that offer a music therapy degree program, check the American Music Therapy Association (AMTA) website and conduct a search. The website also provides an option for you to post a job announcement. Begin your search at www. imnf.org/mhp-book-resources. Another resource is the Certification Board for Music Therapy. Visit the website and follow the procedure for requesting contact information for music therapists in your area, at www.imnf.org/mhp-book-resources.

Below are suggestions on what to expect, and what to look for, when interviewing candidates for a music therapy position. In addition, of course, you will want to explore your candidate's interests and experience with specific patient populations.

## Recruiting a music therapy consultant and/or trainer

To recruit a music therapy consultant or trainer, the search committee will reach out to music therapists (or music therapy practice groups) who have experience in working with organizations like yours; for example, providing staff music therapists, and/or supervising music therapists or music therapy interns.

As you review resumés and interview candidates, here are some qualifications, with plus points to look for:

- Experience as a music therapy consultant to small and large senior healthcare organizations/agencies; deep familiarity with residential and healthcare services, including long-term or nursing home care, inpatient/outpatient rehabilitation, home care and adult care services, and (if relevant) independent and assisted living. *As evidenced by breadth of work experience and ability to highlight successful outcomes, as well as lessons learned.*

- First-hand knowledge of common administrative practices of healthcare organizations/agencies, including clinical administration practices. *As evidenced by breadth of work experience, and supporting references.*

- Understanding of the leadership structures of healthcare and other public service organizations; the different constituencies of these organizations; and the way such organizations are typically governed, managed, and funded. *As evidenced, for example, by having served as a founder, or executive or assistant director, or a member of the board of directors of a healthcare or community organization.*

- Leadership in the field of music therapy, in their area of interest. *As reflected in leadership posts in professional organizations, presentations at conferences, participation in panels addressing important issues, and so on.*

- Willingness to engage in "dialogue across disciplines," to facilitate communication and working relationships with colleagues in clinical and rehabilitation specialties, as well as "arts in health" advocates and educators. *As evidenced by work history, and expressed interests.*

For training, specifically:

- Teaching experience, and knowledge of education methods and practices (pedagogy); ideally, experience conducting in-service trainings for healthcare workers. *As evidenced by work history, samples of workshop materials and evaluations, and possibly videos; also indicated by adjunct teaching positions at a university or geriatric education institute. And don't overlook the experience gained by teaching music performance or composition, as many music therapists do this at some point in their careers.*

- Supervisory experience, as a supervisor of music therapists or music therapy interns in a healthcare setting; or as a supervisor of a training program. *As evidenced by work history and supported by references.*

- Excellent communication skills, and an ability to relate to people of diverse backgrounds and education levels. *As evidenced in interview and supported by references.*

## Recruiting a music therapist (as a full- or part-time staff member)

You can expect that a certified music therapist (MT-BC) will demonstrate the following music competencies, among others (adapted in part, and with some liberties, from Bruscia et al., 1981):

- Professional competence in keyboard and guitar (required), and percussion; and advanced training in the person's primary instrument, or in voice. Ability to play and accompany oneself in a basic repertoire of traditional favorites, folk songs, and popular songs from the cultural and ethnic groups represented in the US population. Make sure that your candidate has a strong background in the music traditions of the communities you serve.

- Experience in leading rhythmic activities and therapeutic drumming circles; ability to play a wide range of percussive instruments (e.g. recorders, bells, gongs, tone bars), as well as one or more melodic or orchestral instruments.

- Basic proficiency in music improvisation, songwriting, and composition. For example, ability to compose songs with simple accompaniment; to elaborate or vary a song or accompaniment, on the spot, to achieve therapeutic goals.

- Ability to express self through movement or dance, and lead others in moving expressively to music.

- An understanding of the dynamics and process of therapy groups. Experience in leading group discussion around thoughts and feelings that are triggered by a shared music experience, to achieve therapeutic goals.

- Experience in leading music listening activities and using recorded music to achieve therapeutic goals.

A certified music therapist will also have numerous competencies that are not primarily musical. Here are a few important qualifications that might be explored in an interview:

- Ability to view another person's world from that person's perspective: this translates into being able to view the patient's or client's world from their perspective, and the family care partner's world from theirs, when providing therapy and care. If you identify this ability in your candidate, it means that candidate will be able to understand your needs, too—which should come across in the interview.

- Capacity for being a team player, willing and eager to work in collaboration with the clinical team; to learn from others, and share skills and information in turn.

- An enthusiasm for supporting patients at all musical and ability/mobility levels; an ability to provide musical experiences that motivate patient participation.

- Ability to communicate well with patients, family, and team members regarding a patient's experience and progress.

- Experience in data collection and analysis.

- Familiarity and comfort with music technologies that support music therapy practice.

## Developing a training program

No one training curriculum will meet the needs of senior healthcare and service organizations when it comes to incorporating music therapy best practices. Training must take into account the specific goals of the organization—the target population, the challenges of integrating music therapy best practices into existing services, and, of course, the resources available.

In current practice, most training programs in music therapy best practices focus on dementia care. They are designed for CNAs, HHAs, and family care partners—those who provide *everyday care* to people with dementia, in residential and home settings. Some trainings may also explore the therapeutic uses of music in dementia groups (where people with dementia may play rhythm instruments together, and take part in social interactions), or in special programs, such as choral groups for people with dementia and their care partners. The increasing use of music in dementia care is exciting, for what has been achieved, and as an indication of what is possible.

**We envision a time when music therapy best practices will inform all aspects of dementia care, as well as care for people with neurologic and mental health challenges, and services for seniors in pursuit of wellness and growth. This guidebook reflects that vision.**

## The framework for a successful training program

Whatever the scope or goals of your training program in music therapy best practices, we recommend that it includes these elements (which are incorporated in this guidebook):

### 1. Introduction: "About you"

Start where your participants are. Your goal is to increase the awareness and understanding of the potential of music to affect patients, so ask participants, "How does music affect you—physically and emotionally?" Ask, for example, "Where (and when) do you generally listen to music?" "What do you experience in these situations?" (For example, a lift in spirits, or improved mood; relaxation, better performance in social settings, etc.) "What is your go-to music when you are feeling down, blue, or depressed? When you like celebrating life? When you just want to be entertained?" *For ideas on how to engage participants through their personal experiences, visit the "About you" features in this guidebook.*

**If possible, arrange for the group to participate in a music intervention beforehand, or as part of the training. Arrange a therapeutic drumming circle or rhythmic activity for the group. Or, if the training will include instruction on using personalized playlists, ask participants to create their own playlists and experiment with using them.**

As part of your introduction, you will assure participants that **no previous music experience is necessary to succeed in using music in patient care**. However, in order to customize your teaching, it would be helpful for you to know about the music backgrounds of participants—for example, how many have played an instrument in school, or sung in a holiday choir; which participants, if any, are active in community music groups, and so on. You might invite participants to share their experiences, or collect this information on a registration form or questionnaire.

## 2. Music and caregiving: Building on what you know

**The introduction will make clear to participants that they already know a lot about the way music affects us, physically and emotionally; and that they use this knowledge, without much thought, in managing their moods, and in other forms of self-care.**

The next step is to help participants discover that they already know how to use music in caregiving. If your participants have ever cared for a child or younger sibling, they probably know something about music interventions. They may have used music to help an infant stop fussing and fall asleep; to keep a toddler happily occupied; to open up a conversation with a preteen. They may have used music interventions in adult relationships as well, singing a well-loved song to comfort an ailing parent or restore communication with a depressed spouse.

Participants in your training can be guided to see how music interventions that are part of family care help shape their work as professional caregivers. Ask participants, "Are there things you just naturally do to establish a rhythm between you and your patient(s), during daily activities?"

## 3. Neurologic foundations: Understanding how and why music interventions work

Participants will benefit from understanding the basis for music interventions, as revealed by clinical experience, music therapy research, and neuroscience, including brain research.

If your training focuses on a specific patient population, such as people with dementia, or people with aphasia and their family care partners, training should begin with a brief review of the salient symptomology of the disorder. How complete and informative this review needs to be will depend on the previous training and experience of your participants. In every case, the presentation should focus on the patient (as a whole person), while highlighting symptoms that are responsive to music, and for which there is evidence that music is an effective intervention.

**The goal is to illuminate the neurological foundation of the disorder, and the way in which music can intervene, alleviating symptoms, and improving health and/or quality of life. For example, understanding brain organization, and the neurological course of dementia, will help participants understand why rhythmic activities work with dementia patients, and why patients in later stages of dementia can often remember the words to familiar songs, but not the names of their relatives.**

**4. How to do it: How to deliver music interventions as part of caregiving**
The goal of training is to provide instruction in, and modeling of, techniques for carrying out music interventions as part of caregiving. **Training will give participants techniques and tips on how to use their voice, the rhythmic movement of their bodies, their music skills, and recorded music, to meet therapeutic goals of the patients they care for.**

Modeling of music therapy techniques is an essential part of the training. For example, arrange for the trainer or staff music therapist to demonstrate drumming techniques and other rhythmic activities that are employed in music interventions. Participants can mirror and then practice these techniques, receiving immediate response and reinforcement.

If your training includes leading groups in rhythmic or song activities, you might introduce role play. Choose participants to play the roles of leader, patient (e.g. dementia patient), and observer. Conduct the activity and provide feedback to the leaders (and patients), with the observers joining in. Closure will summarize learnings from the exercise.

Video presentations designed for teaching purposes are an important tool in demonstrating how music therapists and other team members carry out music interventions. Video support for this guidebook is accessed at www.imnf.org/mhp-book-resources.

**5. The team approach: How to use music therapy best practices collaboratively—with other members of the healthcare team**
To put together a therapeutic music program for dementia patients or other patient populations, you will need administrative support, and practical support for scheduling groups, assigning staff, organizing supplies, and so forth. Most importantly, you will need to collaborate around music interventions that will help the team realize therapeutic goals. How to do this should be addressed as part of your training in music therapy best practices.

**It is helpful to invite key team members to participate in this part of the training.** For example, if you are organizing a therapeutic drumming circle or rhythmic group, to be carried out in part by therapeutic recreation or activities staff, the leadership and staff of these departments can provide valuable advice and perspective. If your training focuses on music interventions for people in rehabilitation, the input of physical therapists or occupational therapists will be helpful. If you are training CNAs, HHAs, or family care partners to use music in everyday dementia care, the director of nursing or nursing supervisor might participate. And if you are planning a group for mental health and wellness in your independent living unit, call on a recreation director or social worker.

## Follow-up

At the completion of training, the music therapist consultant or trainer should administer an evaluation instrument focusing on the objectives and goals of the training; this should be completed by all participants, and the results/conclusions shared with participants and administrative leadership. A follow-up evaluation should be completed in two to three months to measure the effects of the training over time.

Ideally, the training plan will include coaching for trainees as they begin to practice what they have learned, and possibly a refresher course.

In time, an evaluation of the results of music therapy best practices training throughout the facility (or for target populations) will be in order. This might begin with a review of what was happening around the use of music before the institution of music therapy best practices, and what is happening currently. What is different now as a result of the music therapy best practices project? The answers might include references to patient outcomes, as derived from pre- and post-data; references to staff satisfaction and performance; and responses from family members and community.

## Adding musician volunteers to your therapeutic music program

As you implement music therapy best practices, the level of musical activity in your facility will surely increase. You may see opportunities for involving musician volunteers in some of the therapeutic work. As with CNAs and HHAs, musician volunteers can be trained to deliver music interventions that reflect music therapy best practices. There are, however, differences in the training, or guidance, that might be appropriate for a musician. And there are special contributions that a musician volunteer might make to your programming.

Let's look at the basics.

By musician volunteer, we mean a professional or semi-professional musician or singer who has performance experience; or an amateur musician at a comparable level of performance. The musician volunteer might be a career musician who performs in a community orchestra or local jazz clubs, a high school principal who is an avid violinist, a retired minister who was a musician in his youth, or the local mortician who has embarked on a glorious singing career. Yes, these are all real examples. You might be surprised at the number of people known for their success in other fields who are accomplished musicians.

It is helpful if your musician volunteer has connections to your community. Experience of working in intergenerational or senior settings is also a big plus.

In a music-rich environment, musician volunteers already may be regular visitors, performing for patient and community audiences in the lobby and other public areas. These performances might be characterized as entertainment and enrichment activities—and that's all good. Here we are interested in engaging musician volunteers for *therapeutic activities*, as part of a music therapy best practices initiative.

Musician volunteers may conduct or contribute to therapeutic music activities in numerous ways:

- In day rooms, hallways, and common areas where residents congregate.

- At the bedside (one-on-one) when appropriate.

- As group leaders of small groups that offer music-making or listening to people living with dementia, social isolation, and depression symptoms.

- Occasionally, in the rehabilitation gym or other rehab settings where live music has some therapeutic benefit; for example, leading music-making and composition activities for stroke patients or amputees who have limited movement.

- As group leaders and participants in therapeutic drumming circles, dementia choirs, and other music activities involving patients and caregivers.

- As group leaders and participants in special programs that bring musicians together with patients with music skills and interests to play in ensembles, or to compose, perform, and record their own compositions.

Musician volunteers engaged in therapeutic interventions are *not* generally involved in the everyday care of people living with dementia and others who need help in activities of daily living. This means that much of the training in music therapy best practices in everyday care is not directly relevant to them; and yet the uses for music in caregiving may be of interest to musicians who want to understand the foundations of music therapy best practices.

## Contributions of musician volunteers: What you need to know

- Musician volunteers will have music competencies at roughly the level of music therapists—that is, at a higher level than most trained caregivers. (Review the list of music competencies of music therapists above to get a sense of what musician volunteers can contribute.)

- Relatively few musicians are trained as therapists, though many have experience in teaching students with diverse backgrounds and abilities. Like healthcare workers, most have been team players, on teams where individual contributions are well coordinated and highly valued; think ensembles, singing groups, orchestras.

- In the care environment, musician volunteers almost always contribute *live* music (perhaps with technical enhancement or accompaniment) as opposed to recorded music. In this they differ from other non-music therapists, such as recreation therapists and caregivers, who generally use recorded music for therapeutic purposes. Many music therapists believe that music is most therapeutic when it is live.

- Musician volunteers may be able to improvise or compose music in response to patients' moods or feelings in the moment. Music therapists are trained to do this—but it's not a skill that easily can be taught to non-musician caregivers. We should note, however, that musicians are not trained as *therapists*, so they vary in their sensitivity to patients' moods and feelings (especially when feelings are unexpressed). In the best instances, the musician, as artist and performer, is finely tuned to the response of the person who is his or her audience. We should expect that some (not all) musician volunteers will be able to use improvisation and composition effectively in group work or individual interactions.

- Musician volunteers often work well with people who are musicians (or were musicians before entering a senior care facility). For a resident who identifies as a musician, even an amateur, one-on-one time with a musician volunteer may bring moments of extraordinary connection over shared music; increased self-esteem; and the opportunity for creative expression. You may be surprised by the number of residents who have a significant background in music that might be evoked by interaction with a musician volunteer.

### Bringing musician volunteers aboard

At the IMNF, we have had musician volunteers well grounded in dementia and other neurologic challenges, with ideas sparked by music therapy research; and others who went onto the floor not wanting to know the diagnoses of the patients they encountered—grabbing their guitars or keyboards to get to work, communicating through music. Both approaches can work.

The IMNF will include musician volunteers in its trainings. Our strong recommendation is that musician volunteers who participate in therapeutic work have access to the music therapy best practices training that is offered to staff, and to resources like this guidebook; and that they continue to have meaningful access to music therapists who can guide and mentor them, both as therapists and musicians, in the work they do. Our experience shows that musician volunteers welcome this guidance, and put it to use, and that we, as music therapists, benefit from what we learn from musicians who participate in therapeutic programs.

Here are some guidelines for integrating musician volunteers into your therapeutic music activities:

- First, as with all volunteers, musician volunteers should receive an orientation to safety requirements, and policies and procedures of the agency, ranging from legal requirements around protection of patient information to expected behaviors, such as dress code, and security and sign-in procedures. (If you have a robust volunteer program, an orientation will likely be in place to provide this essential information, along with a broader introduction and welcome to the agency.)

- Musician volunteers should also receive an orientation to music therapy goals, especially if a staff music therapist or music therapy consultant has designed the music program that the volunteer will lead. As they work with music-making groups or patients, musician volunteers will need to understand that performance values (so important in the professional life of a musician) are not paramount here. Most volunteers understand this. The music therapist or other staff member should review the summary of music therapy goals (see Module 1) as well as goals for specific patients or patient groups.

- Naturally, music therapists and other staff will give musician volunteers general information on the patient population, to orient them with respect to musical preferences and likely "favorites," and on optimum length of performance for different patient groups.

- When musician volunteers are to serve as group leaders, they should be given an outline of the proposed group format, with timing indicated, and with examples of "hello" songs or introductions, and closing exercise as appropriate (see Module 4). If possible, arrange for the musician to observe a music-based group led by an experienced group leader.

- It is also important to provide practical advice to prepare musician volunteers for issues that may arise. Music therapists must put themselves in the place of the new volunteer and address questions such as "When am I, the performer, finished? What do I do when I'm done playing? What if I'm playing for a comatose patient and the monitor starts to react?" (Wolf & Wolf, 2011, p.32). Another important question that arises in long-term care facilities is: "What if I am playing for people who are in the later stages of dementia and unable to communicate? How can I tell if I am reaching them at all?" Musician volunteers, like recreation therapists and others who use music, should receive training in music therapy best practices.

- Musician volunteers need to know what to do if a song or musical selection causes a patient to burst into tears, or become upset or agitated. This rarely happens—and always unexpectedly. Music therapists (or therapists in general) have a time-tested way of supporting individuals in this situation, in part by acknowledging the person's feelings. Detailed guidance on dealing with unexpected negative responses is provided; guidance to this effect, adapted to your needs, should be provided to musician volunteers. What if the musician is not able to support the patient in this moment? All musician volunteers should know in advance the protocols to follow in requesting support from a music therapist or staff member with mental health expertise, should the need arise.

As you integrate music therapy best practices in your organization, your network of musician volunteers may grow, along with your programming. Consider featuring stories about your volunteers in local news outlets, as a way of attracting interest (and more volunteers) to your music initiatives. It is also a good idea to develop some kind of recognition program for your musician volunteers in your senior care community.

## Orchestras in senior healthcare—It's a trend!

In recent years, top-tier US orchestras have begun to partner with hospitals, healthcare, and service organizations to promote health and wellness for people of all ages. For older adults the focus has been on programs that engage people living with Alzheimer's disease or dementia, and their caregivers.

Driving this trend is the orchestra's mission to make beautiful music, performed to the highest standards, accessible to the widest possible audience. In the past that meant school programs and young people's concerts. Today it also means older people's concerts—and interactive music experiences as well. Generally, these programs are funded by foundation grants.

Examples:

- The Phoenix Symphony Orchestra designed the "B-Sharp Music Wellness: A W.O.N.D.E.R. Project for Alzheimer's" for people living with mild to moderate Alzheimer's or other dementias, as well as their caregivers. Participants regularly attend concerts. They are offered an exclusive pre-concert chat about the day's music with a Principal Timpanist, and have many opportunities to interact with other participants and the world of music.

- The Orpheus Chamber Orchestra, based in New York City, was well qualified to create a program to engage people with Alzheimer's and their caregivers. A chamber orchestra is a small group of musicians, generally with only one person (instrument) to a part. There's no conductor, so the players must keep together by watching and listening to one another. There is a feeling of alert intimacy around this—and this feeling that may be conveyed to others, to the audience, to participants in a group. The Orpheus Chamber Orchestra offers a group program called "Orpheus Reflections," in which musicians play music and interact with people with Alzheimer's disease and their caregivers. Groups take place in small and familiar settings, where group members can feel "close up" to the musicians and the music. This encourages positive social interaction, and sometimes moments of extraordinary connection.

With the growing support for arts in healthcare, we are likely to see growing participation of professional orchestras and ensembles in healthcare facilities, including senior care settings.

What's the takeaway? Orchestras are potential resources for senior healthcare facilities that have established a music-rich environment. It may be that a professional orchestra or ensemble will come to your facility with a special program to support your work, this year or next.

# Music for Mental Health and Wellness

In the early years of Covid-19, we became acutely aware of the high cost of social isolation. People everywhere reported stress, depression, and mental health issues, as "spatial distancing" kept us physically apart from family and friends, colleagues and neighbors. During this time, many of us used music to overcome feelings of isolation and emotional distress.

We will consider the role of music in promoting social wellness during the pandemic in a special section later in the book; and this is an exciting story. (See Music in the Time of Covid: Challenges and Opportunities.). But for now, as we look back at this experience, we have a unique opportunity: and that opportunity is to consider, *with greater understanding than ever before*, what it is like to be socially isolated from day to day, seeing only healthcare "strangers," and hearing voices on a phone. For this is often the experience of older people in senior care settings, and at home alone.

Addressing social isolation and loneliness of patients is a critical responsibility of healthcare providers, because social wellness is a key to overall wellness and health—not just for older people, but for everyone. For this reason, social wellness is where we will begin, in exploring the role of music in promoting mental health and wellness among the seniors in our care.

## Loneliness—and why we need to treat it

For many years, we have known that people with strong social relationships enjoy better health than those with weak social relationships. "Mental health," especially, is thought to depend in part on social factors: having friends, companionship, a supportive family, and connections to the community.

What's just as significant is the effect of social relationships on overall health:

- An analysis of 148 studies with over 300,000 participants from around the world showed that people with strong social relationships are 50 *percent less likely to die prematurely* than people with poor or insufficient relationships (Holt-Lunstad *et al.*, 2010, as cited in Murthy, 2020).

- Amazingly, the impact of social isolation in reducing the life span was shown to be equal to the risk of smoking 15 cigarettes a day, and *greater than* the risk associated with obesity, excess alcohol consumption, and lack of exercise (Holt-Lunstad *et al.*, 2010, as cited in Murthy, 2020).

In other words, weak social connections can be a significant danger to our health.

We must take this into account wherever we provide senior care.


## Social isolation: The risks for seniors

In 2017, the 19th Surgeon General of the US, Vivek H. Murthy MD, made news by declaring that loneliness had become an "epidemic" among Americans of all ages. In 2020, he published a book entitled *Together: The Healing Power of Human Connection in a Sometimes Lonely World* (Murthy, 2020). Murthy had returned to serve the Biden Administration as the 21st Surgeon General of the US. In this role, he was called on to address the ongoing opioid epidemic, the Covid-19 pandemic, and other urgent public health challenges. It is significant that he asked us to turn our attention to the healing power of human connection as we cope with these challenges.

In describing an "epidemic of loneliness," Murthy does not single out older people. Still, older people seem to be especially vulnerable.

In the US, older people are more likely than others to live alone. They are more likely to be widowed; to live in an "empty nest" at some distance from adult children and other family members; to have mobility problems that limit their access to social opportunities.

**Older people in senior care settings are at risk for social isolation**, even though they are seldom alone. Too often the move to a care setting involves a loss of social relationships (and social identity); and the new resident finds themselves among strangers in an unfamiliar environment. A report from the National Academies of Sciences, Engineering and Medicine (2020) notes that 43 percent of Americans over age 60 report feeling lonely.

Healthcare providers and caregivers are most likely to observe the effects of loneliness on the "mental health" and behavior of their patients. **In a long-term care setting, the person who lacks social relationships may present as depressed, anxious, withdrawn, or non-communicative, for example.** What we don't easily see is the impact of loneliness on those chronic conditions and impairments that bring people to long-term care in the first place. One comprehensive review of the research finds that a "particularly devastating" consequence of feeling socially isolated is cognitive decline and dementia (Hawkley & Cacioppo, 2010, p.219). Loneliness is also associated with increased risk of stroke, coronary heart disease, and with "underlying conditions," such as high blood pressure and obesity.

## ABOUT YOU

### Measure your level of loneliness
Take a short quiz, based on the UCLA Loneliness Scale, and adapted by the AARP (2010) to help older people determine their level of loneliness.

**Instructions:** The following statements describe how people sometimes feel. For each statement please indicate how often you feel the way described using the numbers below. *There are no right or wrong answers.*

1=Never 2=Rarely 3=Sometimes 4=Always

1. How often do you feel unhappy doing so many things alone? _____

2. How often do you feel you have no one to talk to? _____

3. How often do you feel you cannot tolerate being so alone? _____

4. How often do you feel as if no one understands you? _____

5. How often do you find yourself waiting for people to call or write? _____

6. How often do you feel completely alone? _____

7. How often do you feel unable to reach out and communicate with those around you? _____

8. How often do you feel starved for company? _____

9. How often do you feel it is difficult for you to make friends? _____

10. How often do you feel shut out and excluded by others? _____

### Scoring
A total score is computed by adding up the response to each question. The average loneliness score on the measure is 20. A score of 25 or higher reflects a high level of loneliness. A score of 30 or higher reflects a very high level of loneliness.

(Loneliness Scale © Dr. Daniel Russell)

**TAKEAWAY**

- How did you score? That is, how lonely are you, as reflected in your subjective rating?

- Does your score suggest the need for any action on your part?

- Do you have patients who would probably score at 30+, reflecting a high level of loneliness?

- Can you think of interventions that might be helpful to these patients?

---

It's clear that we need to prevent and treat loneliness as part of person-centered healthcare. But what does that mean? You can't just write a prescription for "loneliness." *Or can you?*

## Social prescribing

"Doctors are prescribing ways to connect socially for those feeling isolated" is a headline that appeared in the *New York Times*, as part of a series on "The Future of Healthcare" (Hanc, 2021, p.B4). The article describes an emerging approach to health and wellness, in which physicians prescribe interventions or activities that are "non-medical," but likely to improve health outcomes. For example, for older people who feel socially isolated, a physician or healthcare provider may prescribe participation in volunteer work or in social or recreation groups that bring people together in community or care settings. The article focused on social groups structured for people with Alzheimer's disease and Parkinson's disease—both groups in which loneliness is a likely issue. The goal of the activity was to improve quality of life and address health problems, such as cognitive loss and depression, in a social context.

The practice of social prescribing, Dr. Murthy (2020, p.16) writes, "reflects a recognition that loneliness affects our health, and we have a universal need to connect with others." Many of us learned that during the Covid-19 pandemic, didn't we?

## Prescribing music interventions

In Italy, one of the countries hit hardest by Covid-19, neighbors who were isolated in their homes found comfort by singing and playing music from their balconies, in unison. "Music competency is not a requirement, and neither is possessing a traditional instrument," reported *The New Yorker*. "A pot or a wooden spoon can suffice, if only because their sounds will join those of many other people who, from their balconies and windows, are hoping to create a bond through music" (Taladrid, 2020).

In the US, during lockdown, we danced, sang, did yoga together, on online platforms in our own homes.

**Moving rhythmically in time with others brought us together** (even, in this case, when we were spatially apart). This is not surprising: music therapists tell us that one of the best ways of bonding with others is to join a singing group, a rock band, a Zumba class, or some other activity that makes it natural for participants to synchronize their movements. The rhythmic bonding works well with strangers as with others. (Apparently, it also works well on balconies, and over Zoom. And we have known for a long time that it works well in senior care settings.)

In Module 3, we were introduced to music interventions through therapeutic drumming. Mickey Hart, the Grateful Dead drummer (and founder of the wellness organization Rhythm for Life), told us what to expect from a drumming circle in a senior setting: "First, there would be immediate reduction in feelings of loneliness and alienation through interaction with each other and heightened contact with the outside world" (Hart, 1991).

We also learned that "all music-making is social"; that *virtually all music takes place in a social context*; that people can interact with others around music-making, singing, or listening, even when conversation is difficult (for whatever reason). This being so, it is not surprising that music interventions are often prescribed for people who need help in overcoming social isolation.

In this module, we will describe group music interventions that are effective in preventing and treating loneliness, as well as other social or mental health challenges that affect health and wellness.

## Health, "mental health," and wellness: What are our goals?

With encouragement from the US Surgeon General, we have introduced loneliness as a health (and healthcare) issue. That said, most of us are used to thinking of loneliness in terms of "mental health." So it's worth asking, what do we mean by health, "mental health," and wellness?

The World Health Organization (WHO) has defined health as "a state of complete physical, mental and social well-being and not merely the absence

**of disease or infirmity."** This is a broad definition—and enlightened for its time. You might be surprised to learn that it was formulated more than 70 years ago (in 1948, to be exact). The problem is that the WHO definition doesn't work for people who are 70+ today. For most of our seniors, a state of "complete" physical, mental, and social well-being is an impossible goal. So is "merely" the absence of disease or infirmity. Many of us are living past 100, after all.

And then there is the question of what we mean by well-being or "wellness."

Wellness is not the opposite of illness. Unlike "health," which can be modified by degree (e.g. good health, declining health, bad health), "wellness" is always positive and affirmative in connotation. **According to the National Wellness Institute wellness is multicultural and holistic, encompassing lifestyle, mental and spiritual well-being and the environment.** It is a conscious, self-directed, and evolving process of achieving one's full potential. You get the picture.

"Mental health" is a term of convenience, which we will use because it is generally understood and reflects our usual way of thinking. "Mental health" commonly refers to health issues that seem to have no physiological basis but are thought to involve a person's emotions, thoughts, and general ability to adjust to life.

A problem with the term is that mental health is not really "mental" in the sense of being related exclusively to thinking or cognitive processes. And many conditions that we describe as "mental health" have identifiable physical causes, symptoms, and outcomes. (Or might have.) It seems that "mental health" is whatever we say it is. Fortunately, we tend to agree on what we mean.

Here, for reference, is the World Health Organization's concept of mental health; and as you will see it reflects common assumptions and values:

> Mental health is a state of mental well-being that enables people to cope with the stresses of life, realize their abilities, learn well and work well, and contribute to their community. (WHO, 2022)

These conceptions of health, wellness, and mental health are interesting and useful in many healthcare settings. It might be helpful, as well, to come up with a definition of health that meets our special needs as caregivers for a senior population.

What can we say about health and wellness among residents of long-term care and assisted living facilities? And what can we do to make health and wellness happen?

## "Feeling good and functioning well"

Here's a working definition of health and wellness for people who are in senior care settings. A healthy older person is one who is "feeling good and functioning well" (Faculty of Public Health, n.d.). Or as well as possible.

This definition recognizes that it is possible for a person to experience health and wellness even when their day-to-day experience is shaped by chronic illness, impairment, or frailty, or by adverse life events, such as bereavement and institutionalization. What this means is that **a person with a disease or "mental illness" can feel healthy if that person can find—if we can help that person find—a way to balance their strengths and individual gifts, on one hand, against the weight of illness and loss, on the other.**

Coping skills, developed over a lifetime, help older people to experience health and wellness in later life. A responsive environment is also critically important; so healthcare providers and caregivers play a critical role in making the experience of health and wellness possible.

The goal for older people in senior care—and maybe for all of us—is not "complete physical, mental, and social well-being," but the capacity, here and now, to get the most out of life, while leaving the way open for growth, learning, and joy in the future. This involves being engaged in relationships and activities that give meaning to life as it unfolds. In a sense, health is success in living, on one's own terms, in a particular environment.

## Images of health and wellness: "Ask your doctor if this is right for you."

If you watch television, you will have seen a great many images of health and wellness, as personified by people who have chronic and even life-threatening diseases.

The pharmaceutical industry spends billions of dollars a year on advertisements that show people enjoying life immensely, while coping with diabetes, back pain, heart failure, chronic obstructive pulmonary disease, gastrointestinal disorders, cancer, and much else.

We're neither defending nor criticizing these ads—but will note, in passing, that direct-to-consumer advertising of pharmaceutical products is banned in most of the world, and is completely legal only in the US and New Zealand. The ads just might be misleading or inaccurate in the claims they make for medications (and that is a problem).

But big pharma ads say a lot about our ideas about health and wellness. *And that's interesting.* The overarching message is that people with illnesses and health issues can achieve a level of wellness that we all recognize as desirable and attainable. Here's how the message is delivered:

- The person with a significant illness is never shown in bed or resting on the living room couch. All patients are up and about. Heart failure does not prevent folks from venturing forth on European vacations, or taking the boat out. Painful chronic conditions do not prevent people from engaging in white water rafting or vigorous dance. Yes, sometimes a woman (almost always a woman) facing a life-threatening disease will be shown relaxing, with her man on the deck, looking at the beach or the stars, while a large dog wanders into the picture. Or she will be seen extending her arms to her grandchildren, on an open lawn. This woman is not in pajamas.

## TAKEAWAY from the pharma ads
Wellness means being upright, mobile, and ready to engage with others.

- The person with illness or health issues is *almost never shown alone.* This is so, despite the fact that many older people (on multiple medications!) live alone, far from adult children, with minimal social support. The typical subject is shown surrounded by huggable family members of all ages; or gathering with best friends in a robust outdoor setting. Intergenerational camping seems to be a popular activity. If a subject appears alone, he is likely a man in a canoe or kayak. He has our approval.

## TAKEAWAY from the pharma ads
Wellness means being surrounded by loved ones and friends. Illness is not isolating. On the contrary, coping well with illness (taking the medication) leads to social approval and support.

- The person with illness or health issues is seldom shown attending to the routine demands of life. If you have ever been ill or incapacitated for any period of time, you may remember the feelings of wellness that surged when you were, once again, able to do the laundry, the marketing, the family accounts. (How we long to get back to all of it!)

But the images that appear in the ads tend to show people engaged in activities that are freely chosen—recreational and leisure activities, volunteering, and visibly self-fulfilling jobs. Subjects are shown volunteering at food pantries, organizing street fairs, participating in community sports events, or running their own boutique businesses. Or they are having spontaneous fun, as in wandering through outdoor flea markets.

## TAKEAWAY from the pharma ads

Wellness means being free to seek fulfillment in activities of one's choice. Through robust participation in self-fulfilling activities, the ads suggest, a person (on medication) can escape or overcome the constraints that typically accompany illness and the discomforts of age or life in general.

- In line with the above, the person with illness or health issues is often shown (usually very briefly) in a creative activity, such as painting, gardening, arranging flowers, playing the piano, dancing. Even if no such activity takes place, a guitar, or some other symbol of the arts, may well be in evidence. Note that the television is never on in the settings where these creative activities appear to take place. These images of older people engaging in creative activity are no doubt meant to surprise and delight us. (We are not surprised; but delighted, yes.)

## TAKEAWAY from the pharma ads

Wellness means engaging in expressive and creative activities. (Like music!)

- The person with illness or health issues is typically well groomed and attractive, and in evident pursuit of a healthy lifestyle. People of all weights and sizes are shown, vigorously participating in community sports, hiking, climbing and camping, exercising the dog. When food appears, at those farmers' markets and family picnics, the fruits and vegetables tend to steal the scene. As the voice-under intones the contraindications and risks associated with the product, the subjects continue their healthy activities, with exuberance.

**TAKEAWAY from the pharma ads**
Wellness means taking control of your health, by making healthy choices (*and* taking the medication that is right for you).

What's your TAKEAWAY? Do the pharmaceutical ads you see on television generally reflect the ideas of wellness held by most people in the US? Do they reflect your ideas of wellness? Do you think these images have any effect on how people pursue health and wellness in their own lives?

## Music-based groups for mental health and wellness

Music is part of the responsive environment that we hope to create for people who live in senior care settings. In these settings, music for health and wellness is largely delivered in group sessions. Music interventions offered in the group sessions include music-making and singing, moving to music, and listening to music.

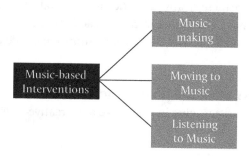

*Figure 1: Music-based interventions*

Music-based interventions include:

- Making music—for example:

  - Playing rhythm instruments, drumming

  - Playing melodic instruments, such as recorders, keyboards, and so on

- Singing, one on one, or in a group or chorus

- Improvising musical rhythms, sounds

- Songwriting

• Moving to music—for example:

- Exercising to music

- Dancing

- Moving to music as part of music-making or listening

• Listening to music—for example:

- Listening to live music, from music therapists and other music partners, including visiting musicians and performers

- Listening to recorded music, on MP3 players, tablets, smart TVs, and phones

Of course, most music interventions involve more than music. A fair amount of social interaction and communication between group members must take place if the group is to achieve its therapeutic goals. Typically, the music therapist or group leader will provide opportunities for sharing and self-expression based on the music experience. This might include:

• discussion of the music, what it means to the group members

• memory work; sharing of personal memories evoked by the music

• storytelling, through music or based on music.

Verbalization or discussion may also focus on:

• the specific health and wellness goals of the group

• ideas for future group sessions.

## Getting started with a music-based group
### Who will attend? Criteria for participation

Music-based groups in senior care settings are generally instituted in response to the needs of the patient population, as identified by healthcare leadership, administrators, and staff. The music therapist works in partnership with other clinicians to establish criteria for participation in the various groups to be offered.

Some groups are very inclusive. For example, a group with a wellness focus might be open to everyone in a certain living unit. Why not? Nearly everyone can benefit from a pleasurable activity that supports creative expression, lifts mood, and enhances self-esteem.

Other groups may require a referral from a healthcare professional. The recreation department is a likely source of referral for patients who are experiencing social isolation or emotional issues. The input of family members and frontline caregivers is also important.

The rehabilitation team is encouraged to refer patients who are receiving therapy for stroke, traumatic brain injury, and other neurological conditions, as well as those who are recovering from hip replacement or other surgery. For these patients, who have experienced a life-changing event, a group that focuses on emotional issues, such as depression, can play a critical role in preventing a decline that leads to extended care.

**The music therapist and other members of the healthcare team will focus on the social functioning, emotional well-being, communication and cognitive abilities, and physical health of a person, in order to place them in a group that focuses on appropriate goals. The therapeutic goals for each person are specific, and described in medical or health-and-wellness terms—not in musical terms.**

Examples of therapeutic goals for an individual might be "To stimulate verbal/nonverbal expressions of feelings," or "To improve interpersonal skills." This might suggest inclusion in a group focused on social and emotional well-being.

### Time requirements

Music-based groups for health and wellness meet at least once a week, in most cases for 45 minutes.

Note that the frequency of group sessions tends to be determined by institutional priorities and resources—not by evidence or guidelines as to what programming may result in the greatest benefit to participants. Evidence suggests that music-based wellness groups that meet more often are more effective in meeting therapeutic goals. In fact, experienced clinicians report that programs should be offered every day for maximum benefit. Even brief interventions, offered daily, have been shown to have a therapeutic effect.

Here's an example. In an IMNF program, in a skilled nursing facility, we enlisted the overhead sound system to play the Macarena on the hour for three minutes, regularly, several times a day—at which time all the staff and residents would engage in the dance. (Picture that—everyone dancing!) This intervention was not part of a research study, just part of everyday care in a skilled nursing facility like most others—*except this skilled nursing facility had music therapy leadership and programming.* And so everyone got a three-minute Macarena break! Did this make a difference? Nursing staff reported an improved mood among patients, as well as reduction in pain and skin lesions that some patients tended to experience as a result of inactivity. (Could it be that the incidence of bedsores is reduced by taking regular three-minute dance breaks?)

Significantly, the WHO suggests that people in nursing homes should have at least 30 minutes of movement exercises every day, within their abilities, along with individualized social engagement. Our experience shows that music powerfully supports both movement exercises and social engagement for people in long-term care.

The recommendation for daily program activity seems equally sound for other senior care settings. When it comes to wellness groups, research suggests that the frequency or "dose" of music interventions has a direct impact on outcomes. As we know, the more regularly we exercise—our minds and bodies and our social skills—the more likely we are to achieve our goals.

## Group size

The size of the music-based group varies, but is usually between four and ten members, with six being the average or optimal number. Therapeutic drumming circles, choruses, and other inclusive groups offered to the senior community may have as many as 20 participants.

## Materials and media

Materials and media required will vary according to the group and its focus. For most groups, the music therapist or group leader will have in hand a guitar, keyboard, drum, or other rhythm instrument. For participants, simple rhythm instruments are often sufficient. (For a list of standard rhythm instruments, see Module 2.)

Music therapists or group leaders may bring sheet music for songs they are prepared to play, or perhaps a songbook they foresee will be useful. Some music interventions may involve handouts, for example lyrics that are to be used as a basis for singing or discussion.

For listening groups, or groups in which part of the session is devoted to listening to recorded music, participants may use MP3 players, tablets, or smart TVs.

## Space

Most groups require a private, contained space that is free from intrusions. Large groups, such as drumming circles, may be held in common, open areas.

## A model: Music-based groups with a focus on social wellness

A music-based group with a focus on social wellness may be recommended for a person who is:

- at risk for, or experiencing, loneliness and feelings of social isolation

- showing deterioration in social skills, including communication skills, due to apathy or isolation

- presenting as withdrawn, or anxious and fearful, in the presence of others

- experiencing a "wall of isolation" in the presence of others due to a life-changing event, or a health issue, such as hearing loss, speech impairment, or memory loss.

For individuals with these and other social issues, the music-based group provides an opportunity to safely share and cope with feelings, fears, and needs.

---

Downloadable HANDOUT at www.imnf.org/mhp-book-resources.

### Basic structure of a music-based group
Welcome piece: hello song

Introduction/recap

Activities and interventions: familiar song(s)

Other music-based activities—for example, engagement with new songs, discussion of lyrics and related themes, moving to music activities, rhythmic and sound improvisations

Live music-making and/or active listening

Closing

---

### The Welcome piece
The group session must have a clear beginning, which we will call the "Welcome piece." Some groups begin with a "hello" song, which helps to introduce group members by name. The music therapist or group leader establishes a rhythm and simple melody, and calls out the name of each participant in turn (or encourages each participant to jump in with their own name). In other

groups, the leader may play a musical motif or group "theme song" to signal that the group is about to begin. For examples of "hello" songs for wellness groups, visit www.imnf.org/mhp-book-resources.

In creating the Welcome piece, the group leader will take into account the cultural and educational background of participants, their level of social and cognitive functioning, and how these factors might affect their expectations. A rhythmic "hello" song can be very effective in bringing together people of all backgrounds, as we see in community drumming circles. Yet it might seem inappropriate ("too much like kindergarten") to group members who come to a wellness group with established notions about therapy, and eager to discuss personal issues with like-minded peers.

Another way of beginning the group is to play familiar music as background, and proceed to go around the group, asking members to introduce themselves and share the issues they've been working on and their expectations for the group. Common issues will likely emerge from the group that will help determine its focus.

## Verbal introduction to group goals

The music therapist or group leader will welcome all participants, noting new members of the group. Some reference to group therapeutic goals may then be offered.

Here are some tips, for verbal introduction and discussion:

- Explain (or refer to) the general purpose of the group in everyday language. Avoid jargon! Do not feel the need to be specific—ideally the goals for the group will emerge in the group itself. Emphasize positive outcomes. That is, you might refer to "making new social connections" as opposed to "overcoming loneliness." Words like "loneliness" and "isolation" will, if relevant, emerge in response to the intentional use of music by the music therapist or group leader, and in group discussion. The goal here is to help participants envision what they will do together, and what they will accomplish. It often helps to accompany discussion lightly, with familiar music.

- If the group has been meeting for some time, review highlights of the group experience in earlier sessions, perhaps calling on participants to give examples or anecdotes. As background, you might play excerpts from music experienced in earlier groups.

- Go around the group and ask members to identify issues that they have been working on and want to discuss. Note: If this has been done earlier, in place of a "hello" song, a recap may be helpful.

A group member may be unable or hesitant to speak up at the beginning of a session, especially when asked to identify a personal issue. The group leader can give the member a pass for the moment, and say something like "That's okay, we'll get back to you," and provide a second opportunity after others have spoken. In some cases, the shy or hesitant member may feel more confident, or be better able to formulate ideas, after hearing from other members.

## Activities and interventions: Familiar songs, familiar music

The music therapist or group leader selects and plays songs based on their strategy for eliciting group discussion and music expression. They give priority to the issue(s) that seem most widely shared or most compelling. In a domain such as social wellness, the issues raised will be general enough for the leader to link participation back to the musical selection.

**The group leader's task is to find out how to process and effectively address the main issue through music.** If the main issue is "feeling isolated," for example, the leader may ask participants about what has made them feel less isolated, less alone, either now or in the past. What activities? What kinds of experiences with friends or colleagues?

The leader will then ask if there is a song or piece of music that expresses group members' feelings or experiences. If no song is suggested, the leader will offer an appropriate song from an internet source; or they might sing, accompanying themselves on the guitar or keyboard. Group members participate by listening, and/or singing along or playing rhythm instruments as accompaniment. Note that if the leader uses recorded songs, this may involve pre-selection of music, or on-the-spot facility with online resources.

### Choosing a song: The basics

In selecting songs for group work, the leader will take into account the age, culture, ethnicity, language, and (if known) the musical style preferences of participants.

The age range of the group tells us where to find music that is likely to be familiar to members. Music therapists have found that **music from a person's adolescence and early adult years is most likely to elicit feelings and memories.** (This is the music that was playing when your group members were likely dating and dancing, falling in love, and getting married.) So the group leader may begin with older songs, such as "You Are My Sunshine," "My Funny Valentine," and "Because of You."

Group members may also have favorites from recent years, especially if they are avid music listeners, or follow particular performers.

Here are some tips for using familiar songs:

- If your group members are in their seventies or eighties, look for songs that were popular in the 1950s and 60s, when they were in their teens and twenties. Do the math. Song lists for different age groups have been developed by music therapists to help you identify the songs that are well suited for your group. Visit www.imnf.org/mhp-book-resources for a list of familiar songs for various age groups.

- Ask group members directly about their favorite songs and golden oldies. No need for anyone to answer aloud, just ask, "What songs do you sing in the shower?" "What would you choose to sing in a karaoke setting?" (*Any stories about that?*)

- Don't assume that group members are living in the past, musically speaking. Ask them about their current favorites—songs and performers they tend to listen to or watch on TV, iPods, or phones; or music events they would most like to attend if given the opportunity. (At the IMNF, our veterans' group for survivors of post-traumatic stress disorder includes a veteran in his mid-eighties who is the first to request songs by contemporary artists.) And by the way, you might generate a lively discussion by asking members what kind of music they "hate," and why.

- Be sure to take into account the diverse cultures and song traditions that may be represented in your group. Song lists for people of different cultures and ethnic backgrounds in the US have been compiled by music therapists to help you meet the needs of your group. Visit www.imnf.org/mhp-book-resources to access song lists for diverse ethnic groups in the US.

### Choosing a song: Therapeutic considerations

In Module 3 we learned that music is a nonverbal form of communication. Music interventions rely on rhythm, melody, and other elements of music to get through to us in ways that words, alone, do not. For this reason, the group leader does not select a song for therapeutic purposes based just on the lyrics (or words).

The music-based group is often recommended for people who are at risk for, or experiencing, loneliness or social isolation. A first thought might be to google "songs about loneliness." But this is not the best strategy. Of course, a song that helps a person express and overcome feelings of loneliness may well be about loss and loneliness ("Hey Jude," "Are You Lonesome Tonight?"). But the song that works is just as likely to be a song associated with friendship, love, or even world peace ("Lean On Me," "Some Enchanted Evening").

What is important is that the song reaches individual group members, helping them feel *an exceptional moment of connection, through the music,* to the singer and others present or remembered. It's a great advantage when the leader can present the song live, looking into the eyes of each group member in turn. Recorded songs, too, may evoke memories or feelings that help a person feel connected to others, and able to sing along and share feelings.

In selecting a song for therapeutic purposes, the group leader must consider the *musical elements* of the song. Here are some guidelines:

- **Select songs that have a melody, rhythm, and tempo that reflects the mood of group members. The music should not be too excitable, or too slow-paced, for the particular group that has assembled on a given day.** The melody may be bright and energetic, calm or consoling, expansive or constrained; and the dynamic level may be loud or soft, depending on the needs of the group as assessed by the leader, through continuous feedback.

  - Group feedback might include body language (*Are members alert or restless?*), level of participation (*Is everybody participating, or not?*), and verbalization (*Are there comments or complaints?*).

- Choose songs that make it easy for group members to sing along and move with the music. **Songs with repetition and refrains are ideal.** The leader can provide the music and lyrics, verse by verse, and group members who may not be familiar with all verses can join in the refrain—singing or chanting, playing a rhythm instrument, clapping, or simply moving to the music.

- Identify songs that lend themselves to lyric alteration—or making up new words around the issues discussed. (An example using "My Favorite Things" appears later in this module.)

### Engaging with music

Music selections are matched to the interests and therapeutic goals of the group. **After a song is played, or listened to, the group leader will engage members in discussing the music and how it relates to the issues they're working on.** For example, when a group member expresses uneasiness in reaching out to new acquaintances, the leader may ask other group members to share times when they experienced similar feelings, and what they did in those situations. The leader may play parts of the song as background or as prompts for discussion.

*Example*:

Suppose the song that is selected is "I Want to Hold Your Hand," by The Beatles. The group member who suggested this song tells the group that he first heard it when he was a freshman at college, feeling all alone, and far from home in an unfamiliar environment. This was a new kind of music, for a new time in his life—and it was exuberant. He remembers that he was shy, maybe withdrawn, and the music helped release some of his inhibitions.

The group leader plays the song, and members join in on its memorable refrains. The leader might then ask the group: How does this song make you feel? (*Happy inside?*) Does it release something in you, as it did for John Lennon? If so, what does this feeling make you want to do? (*Reach out to others?*) How do you expect others will respond? These are questions that might arise from the song, its words, and its music. The leader should ask the questions in an open-ended way, with limited prompting. (The prompts in parentheses are included here so you can see where this might be going.)

Note that in this example it is mainly the music that makes us feel "happy inside." The words never tell us if the singer is successful in holding that hand—and the song (in an alternate version) might have been composed to convey a sense of yearning; but no, we feel the singer's happy resolution in the music, which is achieved through rhythm, melody, harmony, and more. (To see how music conveys the message, try an experiment. Sing "I can't hide," lowering, instead of lifting, your voice on the word "hide." Uh-oh.)

**The group processes the familiar song through verbalization and description of the images and feelings it conveys.** Through engagement with the music, the group approaches its therapeutic goal, which in our example is to overcome feelings of social isolation and reach out to others through shared experiences.

## Music-making: Rhythmic accompaniment

Drumming and the playing of rhythm instruments may be incorporated into just about any music intervention. When the group leader sings and plays a song (or a recording of a song), members can provide a rhythmic accompaniment. Here are some suggestions for initiating a rhythmic accompaniment:

- At the beginning of the group session, make available simple rhythm instruments that are matched to group members' interests and abilities. Invite members to select an instrument (for later).

- After the song (or musical selection) is presented, initiate or demonstrate the rhythm (or invite a group member to do so). The usual way to do this is to accent the first beat (or downbeat) in the group of beats that constitute a musical measure in that particular song.

  In the example above ("1 Want to Hold Your Hand") there are four beats to a measure, so the basic rhythm is 1-2-3-4, 1-2-3-4, etc.). Once this basic rhythm is established, group members may produce this rhythm as an accompaniment to the song, on a hand drum, rhythm stick, or tambourine, for example.

- The group may then go on to express this basic rhythm in different ways. For example, the four-beat framework, or meter, can be filled with twice as many notes, each at half value:

1-and, 2-and, 3-and, 4-and, 1-and, 2-and, 3-and, 4-and

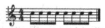

In this case, the drummer is beating faster (with more notes) within the same framework. (That's partly what Ringo Starr does in "1 Want to Hold Your Hand.") Many other expressions are possible. Invite group members to show you *how they feel the rhythm*. In our example, here are some possibilities:

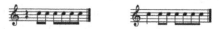

- In some cases, it works to divide the group into "teams" and ask team 1 to play the downbeat, while team 2 plays the rest of the measure; or ask team 1 to play twice as many notes as team 2, within the same measure.

- **Show or model ways in which group members can vary the rhythmic pattern and dynamics to reflect changes in the music.** For example, a slow middle section in a song may suggest fewer beats to be played per measure, or even a suspension of the rhythmic accompaniment. A recurring refrain may suggest dramatic increases in dynamic level. A climactic ending—or a quiet fade-out—will naturally suggest changes in dynamics and/or rhythmic support.

Depending on the music backgrounds and interests of the group leader and members, melodic instruments, such as recorders, flutes, xylophones, and electronic keyboards, may be incorporated into music-based wellness groups.

And the options are greatly expanded in groups that serve (or intentionally recruit) self-identified or amateur musicians.

## Other music-based activities

Music activities that help group members get to know one another can break through walls of isolation or indifference. Below are some activities that are especially well suited for groups focusing on social wellness.

- **Use a blues progression, as background,** to encourage group members to talk about themselves and their lives. (A standard blues progression is a sequence made up of the basic chords that typically appear in jazz compositions, the I, IV, and V chords of a key. You can find many examples on the internet.) First, prompt your group by asking them how they would greet one another if they met on the street. ("What's happening? "How's it going?" "How are you doing?") Ask group members to think about how they might respond to this greeting. Then play a standard blues progression, available on the internet, and demonstrate how this music will help them tell their own stories. Chant spontaneously, and rhythmically, about your own day. ("Today...woke up early...still dark out...did my morning stretches and coffee, waiting for a text to come...then later...") Ask for volunteers to share their day in this way. A standard blues progression for this purpose can be found at www.imnf.org/mhp-book-resources.

- **Use lyric alteration** to change words in a familiar song to reflect something of interest to a group member or the group itself. For example, the song "He's Got the Whole World in His Hands" celebrates everything and everyone that is "in His hands." There are infinite possibilities for group members to add their own examples, reflecting their values, and singing them too.

  The song "It's a Wonderful World" offers similar possibilities. Encourage group members to respond to the song by volunteering their thoughts and feelings about what makes "a wonderful world." The discussion will likely promote social interactions around positive topics. If the leader is able to improvise a verse or two around group contributions, that is a bonus.

  The song "If I had a Hammer" works well with groups focusing on social wellness. First sing the original lyrics, together as a group. Then ask group members, "If you had a hammer—if you had what you need right now, what would you do? Or what would you dream of doing?" This example is drawn from an activity called "Fill in the Blank, MadLib Songwriting," with ideas contributed by Addison

Lucas, MM, MT-BC and Lindi Jane Fogarty, M.M.E.D., MT-BC. Groups can use "fill-in-the-blank songwriting" (or lyric alteration) to share the "likes" of members, in a fun way:

> If I had some chocolate, I'd eat it in the morning, I'd eat it in the evening, all over this land. I'd eat it by itself, I'd eat it with strawberries. I'd share it with all of my brothers and my sisters, all over this land.

> If I had an airplane, I'd fly it in the morning, I'd fly it in the evening, all over this land. I'd fly it to New York. I'd fly it to Mexico. I'd fly it with all of my brothers and my sisters, all over this land.

For more Fill-in-the-Blank Songwriting ideas see www.imnf.org/mhp-book-resources.

- Getting to know someone often involves hearing about their favorite things—their favorite foods, the sports teams they root for, the TV series they watch, and so on. In fact, we typically mention our favorite things in order to define ourselves in a social setting. The song "My Favorite Things," lends itself to expressing (and sharing) one's likes and dislikes. The group leader can pass out the lyrics with blanks where group members can insert their own favorite things, and also what makes them feel sad. The leader and/or group members might choose a theme to help them pull the lyrics together.

*Example:*

Below shows a group "song transformation," of "My Favorite Things" (Abbott, 2018). For the first two verses, the music therapist suggested a theme around "spring and spring flowers." The last two verses provide opportunities for group members to bring up difficult experiences, which no longer seem quite so difficult.

## Song transformation: "My Favorite Things"

Raindrops on *crocus*, And *daffodils and tulips*,
*Bright sunny mornings* and *warm afternoons*,
*Hyacinth* in packages tied up with strings,
These are a few of my favorite things.

Cream-colored *lilies* and *crisp sunny air*,
*Hyacinths* and *forsythia* and *tulips* with *color*,
Wild geese that fly with the Moon on their wings,

These are a few of my favorite things.

When the *neighbor yells*,
When *there's peas for dinner*,
When *I can't get to healthcare*,
I simply remember my favorite things
And then I don't feel so bad.

When *I'm off balance*,
When *I'm in a funk*,
When I feel so *worried*,
I simply remember my favorite things,
And then I don't feel so bad.

*Reprinted with Permission from Barcelona Publishers*

## Movement activities to increase social skills

Moving to music tends to bring group members together.

In the **mirroring exercise**, the leader organizes group members in pairs, and asks paired members to face each other. One member is designated as leader and the other as follower. The leader of the pair executes movements while the follower mirrors or copies these movements (including facial expressions and attitude). Halfway through the exercise, the leader and follower switch roles. Moving together, and paying attention to a partner's movement and gestures, tends to create rapport between participants.

A variation on the mirroring exercise is to ask one member of the pair to execute a movement and the other member to move in an opposite way and manner (with "opposite" physical movements, facial expressions, or attitudes). In this exercise, the second member of the pair has more options with respect to their response, and may feel more assertive; and the first member, or leader, may feel stimulated to respond in turn.

Note that in mirroring exercises the leader's right side corresponds to the follower's left side; so to avoid confusion, the group leader should refrain from offering verbal guidance that refers to "right" or "left."

In a **group member conducting activity**, one member conducts the group in a music activity, such as singing or music-making, or a rhythmic activity such as drumming, or playing rhythm instruments to live or recorded music. The conductor moves their hands, arms, and upper body in a way that keeps the group together. The group switches conductors during the course of the activity, so that each member has a chance to experience the conductor role.

(Note that the music or activity that is "conducted" must be simple enough to require no special skills from the conductor.)

## Closure for the group session

Group sessions should have a clear and satisfying end. Many group leaders choose a song that brings closure, and is repeated at the end of every session. The song might have a goodbye theme ("Happy Trails to You," "Sealed with a Kiss," or "So Long, Farewell" (from *The Sound of Music*)); or it may be a song that provides comfort and tranquility—a kind of winding down ("Simple Gifts," "Somewhere Over the Rainbow," "Amazing Grace"), perhaps a lullaby ("Hush Little Baby," "When You Wish Upon a Star"). It works well if the closing song picks up on song-work or themes that have emerged in group sessions.

## Keeping group members engaged

It is sometimes challenging to engage group members over the course of a 45-minute session, especially if members have diverse interests or are at different levels of functioning.

Here are some tips for keeping group members engaged in music-based activities:

- **Maintain maximum eye contact with group members throughout the session.** Look directly at the person who is speaking, or about to speak. Do not neglect to make eye contact with those who are not participating at a given moment.

- Make sure all members are comfortable in the group setting. Are the chairs (and wheelchairs) well spaced to engage full participation? Is anyone sidelined or left out? Can group members see one another? Can everybody hear?

- Know and generously use the names of your group members. Make sure you know the name or nickname each person prefers. Using a name personalizes the interaction, and helps group members get to know one another.

- Throughout the session, pay attention to facial expressions, posture, and body language of group members. It is easy to see when members are alert and fully engaged. But be alert to signs of discomfort or distress, such as fidgeting, slouching in the chair, averting one's eyes from the ongoing activity, or being otherwise unresponsive. These are indications that the music or activity should be adjusted or discontinued, as it is not fully engaging.

- **Encourage movement around all music activities, including listening.** You can do this by moving in a slightly exaggerated way as you lead the group in the activity; in most cases your movements will be mirrored by group members. *No one should sit still during a music activity.*

- **Encourage humor when it arises, and laughter when it is shared. Laughter is contagious**—it's a synchronized behavior, like drumming or moving together. When we laugh together, we feel happier and more at ease with those around us, says Surgeon General Murthy (2020, p.225), who points out that rarely do we laugh alone. Jokes and funny stories that arise naturally, and are appropriate, can be icebreakers in any group.

## Facilitating group discussion

Much of what happens in the session is verbal; this includes interactions and discussions that occur before and after music-making or listening activities. Here are some suggestions for facilitating discussions that support therapeutic goals.

- Ask non-leading and non-manipulative questions.
  - Avoid: "Did this music make you feel less anxious about reaching out to others?"
  - Better: "What does this music make you want to do? How did it make you feel?"

- Avoid asking questions that tend to put a group member on the defense.
  - Avoid: "How do you know you can't play an instrument if you've never tried?"
  - Better: "Is there an instrument that you'd be comfortable with, for starters? You can choose, and decide if you want to join in."

- Unless you are a qualified mental health professional, avoid giving direct advice to a group member; keep advice general. For example: A group member who is lonely asks: "Do you think it would help me to sign up for volunteer work?"
  Recommended response approach: "Many people find that helping

others is a feel-good experience on many levels." Or: "Volunteering in your community is often a good way to meet others who share your interests. What do you have in mind?" Follow up by asking others to share their thoughts and experiences.

## The music part

Leaders of music-based groups vary greatly in the ways they use music to achieve therapeutic goals, partly because of differences in training and preparation. It is important that the group leader is able to lead with confidence in "the music part," as in facilitating discussions and movement.

Leaders of a music-based wellness group must be able to sing or access recordings of well-known songs, including the likely favorites of group members. For a group leader, being able to sing and accompany a song, on a guitar or keyboard, is an advantage. Advanced music training or a "good voice" is not a requirement, but the music that is experienced by the group must sound good, so many group leaders rely on internet sources for music support. Here are some guidelines for handling "the music part":

- **If you are not a confident musician or singer, it is best to use pre-recorded songs from internet sources, such as YouTube or Spotify.** You can easily search the internet for songs that are most likely to speak to your group members. (For example, you can go to YouTube to find R&B music or music from the 1980s, or anything else—and the musicianship on offer will be of high quality.)

- **Unless you have musical training (and even if you do) your best option is to make the music you present as simple as possible. Music doesn't need to be complicated to have a therapeutic effect. The music you play should never be so challenging that it distracts from the attention you give to group members.**

- Group leaders who provide live accompaniment to group singing or music-making have several options. As a group leader, you can play the melody only—the same note that group members are playing or singing. This is called an accompaniment *in unison*. A simple unison accompaniment can help make members feel supported, and confident that they are playing or singing the "right" note.

  **Group leaders may add harmony—chords or other notes that support the melody and add depth and richness to the music.** Music therapists often use harmony to improvise around a familiar melody, in response to the needs of an individual or group. Generally, this will only be attempted by a music therapist or an experienced musician.

(See discussion on improvisation, specifically "Taking improvisation one step further," later in this module.)

We use the word "harmonious" to refer to pleasing sounds. Technically, though, harmony occurs when any two tones are played simultaneously or very close together. As you may know from exploring a keyboard, not all tones sound pleasing when played together. Certain combinations of tones produce a sharp or jarring sound that we call *dissonance*. In a music composition, dissonance is intentional; as with other art forms, music reflects the human experience, which is not uniformly pleasant or predictable.

**In music, dissonance creates tension, which is followed by a pleasurable resolution or release, created, again, through harmony. Both the tension and its resolution are experienced by the listener or music-maker, emotionally and often physically. This is in part what gives music its therapeutic power.**

Dissonance may be mild, occurring as expected in the course of a melody; or dissonance may be piercing or disruptive. **As group leader, you should be aware that people vary in their level of tolerance for dissonance** (based, typically, on their past exposure to "modern" music—meaning music that does not conform to traditional harmonic conventions). In choosing selections for listening, you may need to take this into account.

- Music selections, such as "hello" or closing songs, can help shape the group session. **You can also use musical signals to help organize group activities.** For example, use a simple drum beat, a single chord, or arpeggio (a broken chord) to gain attention, or to effect a transition from one activity to another. (This technique is used effectively by preschool teachers, and no less by savvy TV producers who chime us to attention for one segment after another: because it works!)

- Finally, the music part works best when it's clear that the leader is having fun. In the words of a music therapist experienced in working with people at all levels of function, "Remember to command and move the energy, notice the space you are in, and maximize it. And have fun."

## Music-based groups with a focus on mental health and emotional wellness

Music-based groups that focus on emotional wellness are likely to benefit those members of the senior community who want to reach or maintain a state of "feeling good and functioning well"—in other words, just about everybody. Caregivers too. We can all benefit from music interventions that lift our mood, and help us to express and share our feelings in a supportive environment.

**Most of us recognize that the music we listen to affects us emotionally, in the moment. And when we select the music ourselves, the effects are mostly positive.** In a music-based group, the leader plays music, and intentionally engages group members in music experiences that promote emotional wellness *and* address common mental health challenges.

## Music and emotions—what's the connection?

Music has been called the language of emotions. The building blocks of music are not words or visual images, but rather sounds; so, we might ask, what does sound have to do with emotions? What is the sound-to-feeling connection?

Consider an emotionally charged moment in your own life, when you waited for news of a loved one or an important event. "It's so good to hear the sound of your voice," you say, feeling relief before you've even heard the full story. What we experience, in a moment like this, is the "sound-to-feeling connections we have made throughout our lives with the people we care about," writes Nina Kraus, a neuroscientist who has done ground-breaking research on sound and hearing (Kraus, 2021, p.52). The voice—the sound—is a powerful trigger. (*Ask yourself: would you feel the same physical response to a text message on a screen; the same easing of breath, the immediate flooding of warmth throughout your body? Probably not.*)

**Sounds powerfully trigger our memories and engage our emotions.** The reward system in the brain, which is responsible for emotional responses, such as pleasure and fear, and emotionally based motivation and learning, has "privileged access to hearing centers in the brain" (ibid.). This means that a sound message travels through *very fast* neural pathways, immediately triggering emotional responses, before the thinking brain has had time to process the sound event (ibid.).

**The reward system in the brain is closely connected to its hearing centers—so it kicks in powerfully when we listen to music, especially music that we know and love.** Neuroscientists have shown that the pleasurable experience of listening to music releases dopamine, a neurotransmitter that is also released in response to rewards such as food, sex, exercise, and recreational drugs. Listening to music affects blood pressure, heart rate, respiration rate, galvanic skin response, and other physiological responses in ways that indicate emotional arousal.

Leaders of music-based groups use music to meet a wide range of mental health goals. For example, they select music that helps people to:

- incorporate a reliably pleasurable (or positive) experience into daily life

- share a pleasurable experience with others, in a social setting (or virtually)

- manage moods and regulate emotions in daily life

- reduce anxiety and stress

- experience higher energy levels and enhanced vitality and wellness

- improve overall physical function, including fluidity of movement, posture, balance

- reduce distress from low-level chronic pain

- improve mental focus and concentration

- improve confidence and self-esteem

- discover new activities and creative outlets, and learn new skills

- contribute to the community, through music-making, performances, and shared audience experiences.

## Rock 'n' roll but not sex or drugs: A study suggests that music activities were most helpful in coping with emotional distress during Covid-19

Research has shown that music can be an effective tool for managing emotions and reducing stress and depression, both in everyday life and extraordinary circumstances. That being so, a team of researchers was interested in assessing the role of music in helping us to cope with psychological distress during the early acute phase of the Covid-19 pandemic. Their initial findings have relevance for public health efforts in response to the Covid-19 and future pandemics.

In the abstract (or introductory summary), the authors write:

The Covid-19 pandemic has deeply affected mental health. We assessed which of many leisure activities had positive psychological effects, with particular attention to music, which has been reported anecdotally to be important. Questionnaire data from over a thousand individuals primarily from Italy,

Spain, and the USA during spring 2020 show that *people picked music most often as the best activity to cope with psychological distress...* [emphasis added] (Mas-Herrero *et al.*, 2020)

The results may be summarized as "Rock 'n' Roll but not Sex or Drugs"—and better yet in Figure 2, below.

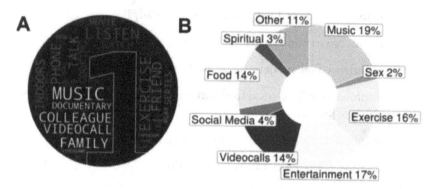

*Figure 2: Helpful activities for coping with Covid-19 pandemic-related psychological distress*

Figure 2 shows that during the period of acute lockdowns in the initial spring surge of the Covid-19 pandemic, music-related activities were reported to be the most useful for 19 percent of the sample. Music involved all music-related activities including composing, playing an instrument, or singing; food included all activities related to cooking, baking, or eating; videocalls referred to talking with family and friends; social media included all items related to the use and discovery of social media applications; exercise covered all activities related to sport, indoors or outdoors; entertainment included watching series, documentaries, and movies, reading books, and listening to the radio; spiritual comprised any religious (e.g. prayer) activity, yoga, and meditation; sex included any sexual or erotic activity.

The Covid-19 epidemic revealed much about the challenges of healthcare, and introduced new possibilities to connect through music. At the end of this book, "Music in the Time of Covid: Challenges and Opportunities" highlights lessons learned, and resources that will help us meet the continuing challenge of Covid-19, as well as future challenges.

# "Musical chills"—intensely pleasant emotional responses to music

Robert Zatorre, PhD, a neuroscientist at Montreal Neurologic Institute at McGill University, has found that:

> Some people seem particularly sensitive to music, showing not only a lot of interest and liking of music, but also displaying physiological responses to music, such as the very pleasurable "chills" (a response involving goosebumps and tingles up the spine). Others never (or hardly ever) experience these intense responses, even though they are self-professed music fans. (Blood & Zatorre, 2001)

Have you ever experienced chills when listening to a highly pleasurable piece of music? Or to music with a strong emotional association?

Matthew E. Sachs, PhD, as a graduate student, conducted experiments at Harvard University to discover what might explain "musical chills" (Sample, 2016). From a group of volunteers, the research team selected a "chill group," and a "no chill group." To confirm that the groups met their selection criteria, they measured the physiological responses of both groups to music they had brought in from a playlist of favorites, and to other music selections that served as controls. Then they monitored the brains of subjects in both groups, using a scanning technique that showed the neural connections between different regions of the brain.

What they found is that brains of people from the "chill group" had more nerve fibers running from the auditory cortex (involved in basic hearing ability) to two other key regions, one involved in processing feelings, and the other thought to monitor emotions.

Zatorre's research had shown that when a person listens to highly pleasurable music, the auditory system is strongly coupled to the brain's emotion and reward systems. The results of the "musical chills" study suggests that people who experience "chills" from music have a stronger connection than others between the auditory and emotion systems in the brain. We don't know if learning or experience accounts for these brain differences.

## TAKEAWAY

Music that is extremely pleasurable to us increases the releases of feel-good chemicals in the brain. Make a playlist of the songs that have this very positive effect for you, and consider making it your "go-to list" when you need an emotional lift. Similar playlists can be made for the people you care for, to help improve their mood.

## Applications in senior care settings

We've said that just about everyone can benefit from a music-based group that focuses on emotional wellness. In a senior care setting, though, groups tend to be recommended mainly for people who are *not* feeling good or functioning well from day to day, due in large part to emotional (or "mental health") issues.

## Who will attend? Criteria for participation in groups with a mental health focus

In order for a person to be referred to a music-based group with a mental health focus, they must usually meet the criteria established by the health-care team. Criteria for referral generally focus on the type and *severity* of the person's emotional problem. For example, depression symptoms are common in care settings (as elsewhere). In making a referral, the healthcare team will need to assess whether a person is experiencing a run of bad moods, or a full-blown depression.

As we know, emotional problems often arise due to a specific situation. In many cases, an older person experiences depression symptoms in response to a recent bereavement, an illness, or a loss of social connections on transition to residential care. Or a person may have a tendency toward mild depression, or a melancholy temperament. In other cases, emotional problems are long-standing and of deeper significance to a person's health and well-being. Examples of these more serious health challenges include major depressive disorder, bipolar disorder, anxiety disorders, such as phobias, and PTSD, among many others.

**Music therapy has been shown to be effective in treating people across the mental health spectrum. That said, in senior care settings the criteria for participation in a music-based group will exclude those with serious psychiatric disorders.** People diagnosed with serious disorders are treated by mental health professionals, including board-certified music therapists, and mostly in individualized sessions. When group music therapy is offered to people with serious mental health problems—as it may be for veterans and other peer groups with PTSD, for example—the group leader should be a music therapist with experience in treating the disorder. What this means is that leaders of music-based groups in senior care settings are not providing therapy to people with serious mental health problems. They can be confident in offering music interventions that address the therapeutic goals of participants who are referred to the group.

## "Depression" or depression symptoms

The most common mental health challenge among older people is depression, in its many forms. It's a challenge that most of us are familiar with.

People often say that they are "depressed," meaning, in most cases, that they have "depression symptoms," such as prevailing feelings of sadness, lack of energy, excessive worries, and trouble concentrating.

When depression symptoms persist, resulting in significant distress and an inability to function well in important areas of life, a person may be diagnosed with *depression*—mild, moderate, or severe—with reference to specific medical criteria. This assumes that a diagnosis is made; unfortunately, depression is often undiagnosed and untreated among people of all ages.

Among older people who are coping with physical illness and cognitive decline, depression symptoms are common: for stroke survivors, and people living with Parkinson's disease, heart disease, or dementia, depression is often part of the larger picture. Even so, the rate of treatment for depression and other mental health issues is low. One summary of research in this area found that between 50 and 75 percent of residents with depression in long-term care nationwide were receiving no treatment for depression (Dow, 2011, as cited in Clemons, 2021).

## Who is depressed?

CDC data shows that older people are not more likely than other adults to experience severe symptoms of depression. However, people over 65 (as well as those between the ages of 18 and 29) *are* more likely to experience *mild* depression. These CDC findings are based on the administration of the eight-item Patient Health Questionnaire depression scale (PHQ-8), in which sample adults were asked how often in the past two weeks they had been bothered by the symptoms, such as: "Little interest or pleasure in doing things," "Feeling down, depressed, or hopeless," "Feeling tired or having little energy," "Feeling bad about yourself, or that you are a failure, or have let yourself or your family down." Answers are summarized into scores that indicate no or minimal symptoms, or mild, moderate, or severe symptoms of depression (Kroenke *et al.*, 2009). (Access the Patient Health Questionnaire depression scale (PHQ-8) at www.imnf.org/mhp-book-resources.)

Using this methodology, the CDC found that the past two weeks, 21.8 percent of women and 15 percent of men over the age of 65 had experienced some degree of depression—mild, moderate, or severe. More than half of those studied—about 12 percent—experienced mild depression (Villarroel & Terlizzi, 2020). Other reporting by the CDC suggests that depression in general is higher among older people who require home healthcare or are cared for in hospitals or institutions. It follows that mild depression is higher among older people in long-term care settings.

**The truth is that we don't know how prevalent depression is among older adults in residential care.** Even before the pandemic, one estimate of the "prevalence of depressive symptoms" in this population was as high as 44 percent (Clemons, 2021). Other studies, depending on their measurement tools and other factors, reported lower estimates. It's hard to know: depression symptoms among older people in residential care are mixed up with (or show high rates of comorbidity with) other illnesses. Mild depression may slip through the cracks, so to speak.

### What do you think?

**On any given day, how many of your patients seem to be experiencing depression symptoms?**

What percentage of those you care for are almost always in a sad or non-responsive mood, lacking energy or interest to participate in daily activities?

How about 50 percent? The CDC (2014) has reported that depression affects nearly half of all nursing home residents in the US. The larger estimate probably reflects the experience of many CNAs and other healthcare providers, because they see depression symptoms among many of the people they care for, every day. And when they see these symptoms, they feel a need to do something about it.

### Music-based groups with a focus on reducing depression symptoms

In describing the music-based group for emotional wellness and mental health, we will focus largely on therapeutic activities that reduce common depression symptoms.

**Depression, as a mental health illness, should only be treated by mental health professionals, including music therapists. At the same time, we can't ignore the fact that CNAs and other caregivers often care for patients who are sad and withdrawn or have other depression symptoms. Experience shows that caregivers who are not music therapists or mental health professionals can provide music listening or music engagement that can lift a patient's mood, and encourage activity and social interactions that will decrease depression symptoms.**

### Depression symptoms: A closer look

Depression is characterized by two main features:

1.  **Depressed mood, most of the day, nearly every day.**

2. **Markedly diminished interest or pleasure in all or most activities.**

Other symptoms associated with depression include:

- Significant weight loss when not dieting, or weight gain; or decrease or increase in appetite.

- A slowing down of thought and a reduction of physical movement (observable by others).

- Fatigue or loss of energy.

- Feelings of worthlessness or excessive or inappropriate guilt.

- Diminished ability to think or concentrate, or indecisiveness.

- Recurrent thoughts of death, recurrent suicidal ideation without a specific plan or a suicide attempt, or a specific plan for committing suicide.

To be *diagnosed* with major depressive disorder, or clinical depression, a person must experience *five* or more of these symptoms, nearly every day during the same two-week period, and at least one of the symptoms should be either 1) depressed mood or 2) loss of interest or pleasure in all or most activities (Truschel, 2022; American Psychiatric Association, n.d.).

As noted, the participants referred to a music-based group in a senior care setting are unlikely to have been diagnosed with serious mental illnesses, such as severe depression (major depressive disorder). That's because very few senior care institutions have an on-staff or consultant music therapist. (It is our hope that this will change in the future.)

For members of a music-based group, **music is uniquely powerful in reducing the two main symptoms of depression at all levels—a depressed mood, and loss of interest and pleasure in activities of daily life.** These symptoms are common among older people in all care settings. Music therapists are committed to sharing their knowledge and skills with other health professionals and music partners, so that senior care communities can offer music-based groups widely, to everyone who will benefit.

## Reaching people with depression symptoms

**One of the reasons that music is effective in reaching people with depression symptoms is that** *music is a nonverbal form of communication.* Music can get through to us and change the way we feel, *even when words are ineffective.*

If you've ever tried to simply talk a person out of a depressed state, you probably know that this is not a winning strategy; nonverbal communication is more likely to get through. This includes not only music but other nonverbal persuasions—a hug, a touch on the arm, the mute attention of the family dog, the timeout for a cup of tea, and so forth. The expectation is that music and other forms of nonverbal communication will make it more possible for a person with depression symptoms to begin to respond to others, in nonverbal ways (e.g. moving with and sharing music), and then by talking. That is often what happens in a group setting.

**Music-based groups that focus on emotional wellness follow the basic structure we have presented earlier in this module, and utilize many of the same techniques—familiar songs, rhythmic activities, music-making, and discussion strategies to encourage communication and self-expression.** Here we will present additional strategies for engaging and motivating people with depression symptoms—for this is often a challenge to group leaders.

In a music-based group, the leader's task is to find out how to process and effectively address the main issue through music. **If the main issue is feeling depressed, or "blue," or "down most of the time," this presents a challenge to group activity, as such.** Among the symptoms of depression are a slowing down of thought, reduced physical movement, and fatigue or loss of energy. These symptoms, as well as loss of pleasure and interest in usual activities (which may have included music), are typically reflected in lack of interest or response from some group members, especially in early sessions.

### What is a group leader to do?

Here are some tips and strategies for reaching non-responsive group members:

- Perhaps you've offered a song, or put forward a discussion question, and there isn't much response from one or more group members. Don't assume that this is a failure on your part. **A lack of *verbal* response does not mean that a person is unresponsive to the music, or to your discussion prompts.** Do not insist on a verbal response if it is not forthcoming. Focus on the music and on other forms of nonverbal communication. Among the nonverbal cues that are working for you in the moment are eye contact, nods, smiles, and body language, and the presence or nearness of other group members who are leaning into the music and the activity.

  **Experienced music therapists know that you can begin an individual or group session, by playing a rhythm, or singing a song, *without making any demands*. The music, itself, is a kind of gift, with its unspoken values of sharing and caring.**

- When some members are slow to respond, or seemingly unresponsive, group leaders often turn to other more responsive members to help carry the group forward. (We've all seen teachers who do this, always calling on the student with the raised hand.) Within limits, this is okay: those more active members are responding to the intervention that is offered, from which they stand to benefit; and their participation in the intervention may encourage others to respond, to their benefit as well. As group leader, you can continue to include non-participating members in the activity, by maintaining eye contact and by calling on all members by name in the course of the activity.

- It's important to remain engaged and naturally upbeat throughout the session. Group leaders should acknowledge all participation in a positive way, even if participation is little more than attendance, or being present. Attendance is good! You go from there.

## Music interventions that focus on depression symptoms

Below are discussion prompts, activities, and suggestions for leaders of music-based groups that focus on depression symptoms. Discussion prompts may be adapted for use by family care partners.

- The group leader might begin by asking participants to think about their experience with "good moods" and "bad moods" in their own lives. How would they describe "bad moods?" Responses might include references to feeling "blue," "downhearted," "depressed."

- Ask group members if they can think of a time when they felt more upbeat, more positive than they do right now, this week, over the last few months? Do not be concerned if there are no *verbal* responses to this prompt. Look for nonverbal cues and body language to tell you if group members are responding.

- Go around the group and ask, "What factors or experiences seem to influence your mood (or other people's moods), one way or another?" For depressed moods, answers will likely focus on health issues, losses and bereavements, loneliness, disappointments, personal or family failures, financial distress, and so on. For positive moods, answers will likely be less specific. **Try to help members capture images and memories that they associate with positive moods and feelings of wellness.**

  Avoid asking participants directly if they are depressed, and why. Especially at the beginning of the session, participants may not feel comfortable, or able, to talk about a depressed mood or the reasons for it. Or they may not be able to acknowledge their feelings. **Use prompts and questions that encourage participants to speak, at**

**first, in general terms; this provides openings, as well, for those who are not ready to share personal experiences.**

- **Many people use music to help manage their moods**—and this has applications in group and individual sessions. Often when we select music to listen to, we are engaging in a form of self-help—*matching the music to the way we want to feel* in the next few minutes, or more (MacDonald, 2013). Ask group members (or your loved one) how they want to feel five minutes from now. Ask, "What's one word to describe the mood you want to be in for the rest of the hour?" Not everyone will respond verbally, but it's likely that those who respond will be met with a silent consensus.

  Bring up the concept of the personalized playlist (see Module 5). If group members have developed their own personal playlists, that's great: if not, ask them to imagine (or write down) their selections.

- Ask group members for examples of the music selections on their playlists that would enhance their feelings of wellness (make them feel better). Specifically, ask, "What songs or music selections can be relied on to improve your mood, when you are feeling blue/sad/depressed?" (And what about right now?)

- Choose a song from one of the playlists, calling on suggestions from group members. Find a recording of the song on your phone or computer, and play it for the group.

- Encourage group members to participate by listening actively. Engage them from the outset: announce the selection, and perhaps suggest what they should listen for. Encourage members to sing or hum along if the song is familiar to them.

- Move in a slightly exaggerated way with the music, or initiate foot tapping or some other rhythmic movement. The goal is to keep members alert and moving with the music.

- As follow-up, offer additional selections, drawn from the group (or alternately a song that you have prepared for this purpose). After group members listen to a song (maybe more than once), ask them what mood or feelings the music conveys to them. Encourage discussion of individual responses. Play parts of the song as background and prompts to discussion.

- Choose music that has the potential to enhance group mood over the course of the session. Music therapists have found that one way to use music to relieve depression is through interventions that incorporate progressively more stimulating music (Clair, 1996). In a group, this might mean choosing music that matches the mood of group members on entry, then introducing brighter, more stimulating music as the group progresses toward therapeutic goals.

For example, if the group mood feels subdued and unmotivated, begin with music in a slow tempo and steady rhythm, and perhaps a somber tone. Ask group members to breathe along with (in time to) the music. Then introduce music with a slightly faster tempo; again, ask group members to breathe with the music; perhaps introduce a gentle exercise, such as raising the arms in time with the music ("conducting"), and/or bending the knees with the beat (the dance step called plié, pronounced "plee-AY"). Follow this with faster and brighter selections, including music with syncopation. Encourage group members to move to this fast-paced, stimulating music. Group members who must remain seated or in wheelchairs can move their arms or feet in time to the music.

## ABOUT YOU

### Music and mood management. What works for you?

Most of us use music to manage our moods on an everyday basis. "Every time we select a piece of music to listen to, we make a number of very sophisticated and highly nuanced psychological assessments about our current state of mind and the environment in which we are listening to music," writes R. MacDonald (2013), in a review of music, health, and well-being. We choose what we need, without much conscious effort.

In this questionnaire we invite you to take a minute to think about the music you use to manage your moods under different circumstances. Fill in the blanks with a general description of the music that works for you (e.g. "folksongs" or "ballet music"), or the names of specific music selections, composers, or performing artists or groups (e.g. "songs by Peter, Paul and Mary/Puff the Magic Dragon" or "ballet music from Tchaikovsky/Swan Lake or Sleeping Beauty"). If you can, say (or think about) *why* this music has the desired effect. (Is it the melody, the lyrics, a specific memory or association evoked by the music?)

Enter your responses below:

1. When I don't feel well (when I am in bed with a flu, or aches and pain), my go-to music is:

2. When I begin to feel overwhelmed by tasks and responsibilities, the music that helps me keep calm and carry on is:

_____

3. When I simply need to relax, at the end of a busy or tense day, my go-to music is:

_____

4. When I need courage to deal with uncertainty, the music I turn to is:

_____

5. When I feel down, blue, or depressed, the music that is most likely to lift my spirit is:

_____

6. When I feel like celebrating life, when I am thankful, or surprised by joy, the music that expresses my state of mind is:

_____

## TAKEAWAY

Your patients bring to their current situation their own go-to music—often on personalized playlists that can be accessed on phones or other digital devices. Their go-to music, like yours, is potentially therapeutic: it can be used (by you and others in the course of caregiving) to help them manage their moods and anxieties. There is evidence too that listening to preferred music can reduce a person's perception of pain in some situations.

## Dealing with unexpected emotional responses

In a music-based group for emotional wellness, one of our goals is to use music to improve mood. There is a growing evidence base to support the use of favorite songs (and personal playlists) in promoting emotional wellness in people at all levels of functioning. But personal playlists are, well, personal. What happens if a familiar song, presented in a group setting, has an unexpected effect on an individual member, for personal reasons that you are not in a position to anticipate?

**In other words, what should the group leader do if a specific music selection brings forth sad memories or feelings—even tears—in one of the group members? What if a group member becomes upset or agitated on hearing a song or musical selection?**

First of all, the group leader should focus totally on the needs of the person who is affected, and not berate or blame themselves for this unexpected response. (It's not about you.)

Second, the leader should put the response in context—which may well show that it is not so negative or harmful as first appears. Sadness is a legitimate human emotion, and as such it may be evoked by music. In our individual lives, memories of sad events or times of unhappiness may be evoked by particular songs and musical selections. When this happens to an individual in a group setting, the role of the leader is to help that person feel, express, and share their sadness in a way that is therapeutic for them. Perhaps the group member was unable even to feel their sadness before coming to the group; and so they were not able to express it. Perhaps their response, now, is a moment on the way to emotional healing.

The leader can begin by acknowledging the emotion: "I know this is really sad for you," and by offering an opportunity for emotional sharing: "Tell us why"—and if that is difficult, "We will help you. You know, we've been sad too." Now that the emotion is expressed (and maybe shared), the leader is in a position to give direct and meaningful comfort, in a social context.

The leader should take a minute or two, after the interaction, and then suggest, "Let's move to another song"—not because there was anything wrong with the last song, or the way it was experienced—but because the group members can continue to interact around songs that awaken them emotionally and in other (sometimes personal) ways. It often works well if the group member who experienced the sad emotions is able to suggest another song.

In rare instances, a group member, on hearing a song, may become upset or agitated in a way that makes it difficult for them to participate in the group or return to daily activities. The leader should help the agitated person to find comfort within the group, as suggested above; and if it seems that more support is necessary, the leader should follow protocols to request support from healthcare providers who focus on mental health issues. Group leaders should have a clear understanding of the mental health resources that are available for the patients they care for, in case unexpected needs arise.

## Moving to music to reduce depression symptoms

Richard A. Friedman, MD, a leader in the treatment of chronic depression, says that "Exercise is the first step for all my patients. It boosts everyone" (Solomon, 2015, p.138). In fact, **exercise is strongly recommended for people with depression symptoms, from mild to severe.**

Depression symptoms include a slowing down of thought and physical responses and a loss of energy. People who are sad or withdrawn may feel sluggish and dull; to others they may appear lacking in motivation. They are aware of the need to "get off the couch," to "get the blood flowing," if only they could do so. Exercise is often prescribed.

Exercise "boosts everyone," in part because it produces feel-good neurochemicals in the brain—including endorphins, such as dopamine and serotonin. These neurochemicals work to improve mood, while helping us to flourish physically, within the limits that age, illness, or disability may impose on us.

Regular exercise, as prescribed by a health professional or coach, can improve or maintain cardiovascular and respiratory function, help prevent loss of muscle strength and bone loss, and improve balance and coordination (preventing dangerous falls) among many other benefits. In older people, regular exercise helps slow the loss of brain volume, which may help prevent age-related memory loss and cognitive decline (Reynolds, 2021).

**The problem is that people with depression symptoms are often unmotivated to exercise.** That's where music comes in. **In healthcare settings, and elsewhere, it has been shown that people are more likely to enjoy exercise, and to stick to an exercise program, if they exercise to music.** That may be because music produces those feel-good endorphins that make us want to take that last lap.

In a music-based group that focuses on depression symptoms, an immediate goal is to awaken the person, both body and mind, to a healthy, invigorating experience, here and now; and this is often achieved by moving, as in moving forward.

## Leading exercise activities in groups for people with depression symptoms

- **As group leader, take every opportunity to move about, spontaneously and naturally, throughout the session.** Provide cues that help members move to the music—slightly exaggerating your own movements: for example, with a nod and a flourish, extend an open hand toward group members to invite participation. Walk about; add dance steps if that feels natural.

- **Create situations in which group members must move in order to participate fully.** For example, introduce physical movements during a listening experience (clapping or swaying, or playing a simple rhythm instrument). Offer activities in which group members change or rearrange their chairs; arrange things so that members need to move about in order to access an instrument. Be sure to include movement options for group members who must remain seated, but who can participate with head, torso, arm, and leg movements.

- **If you choose to incorporate music-based exercise into a group focused on emotional issues, it often serves well to collaborate with a recreation therapist. A dance therapist, if available, is also a valuable collaborator.** Be clear about the therapeutic goals established for your group, and the context for exercise or movement activities. A collaborative approach will help identify music-based exercises well suited to your goals, as well as tips and techniques that reflect experiences across disciplines.

Here are some music-based movement activities for you to consider:

- **Ask group members to act out movements from their lived experience**; for example, sports movements, like the swim crawl, or strokes from golf, baseball, or tennis, or movements involved in driving, gardening, or housework. (You might initiate the exercise by providing an example from your own life—for example, demonstrating the movement involved in playing a musical instrument or leading a chorus.) As group members act out familiar movements, provide a rhythmic background to support and extend the exercise; a rhythmic accompaniment will also encourage others to join in, by imitating the movement, or by nodding, tapping feet, and so on. Ask questions that encourage discussion of moods and memories associated with these movement-modulated experiences.

- **Select recorded music that is rhythmic and dance-like, taking care to match the energy level of the music to the energy and mood of the group.** Your goal will be to encourage movement that improves mood and alleviates depression symptoms. In most cases, you will begin with music that is slow to moderate in tempo, and not overly stimulating at the outset. The music you choose is very likely to reach a high point, or build toward a climax in form or feeling at some point. Through the music, group members will experience this movement toward heightened feeling—and the resolution that follows. This experience will be reflected *in their physical movements, and in the emotional domain.*

- Invite group members to move freely to recorded music, while imagining a scenario of awakening and growth. For example, group members might imagine that they are seeds growing into sunlight, or trees with branches reaching toward the sky. Some group members may feel self-conscious or uncomfortable with this imagery, in which case they might simply do stretch and bending exercises to the music.

  - Music selections that work well for awakening exercises include: Faure, Après Un Rêve, Op. 7 No. 1; Elgar, Chanson De Matin; Grieg, Morning Mood from *Peer Gynt Suite*, Op. 45; Rossini, Call to the Cows from *William Tell Overture*; Borodin, Polovtsian Dances from *Prince Igor*; and Pärt, Spiegel im Spiegel.

  - Another option might be to ask group members to "freeze" in their position in their chairs, remaining completely immobile until an impulse leads them to "unfreeze" (awaken, come alive) and move with the music (or until you or another group member signals them, or invites them to begin moving).

- For additional insights and suggestions, review the "movement to music" content that appears throughout this guidebook, including music-based exercises developed for people with dementia; for people undergoing rehabilitation after stroke or other injury; and for those in treatment for chronic or progressive diseases. These exercises may be adapted for groups that focus on emotional issues. As we have seen, rhythmic activities and many other music interventions are inclusive, and can be adapted to meet the needs of people at all levels of functioning.

  - For example, stretching motivates movement of different parts of the body. Stretching exercises may also help people with depression symptoms become active, lift their shoulders, look around, and achieve a more erect posture, in line with therapeutic goals. (As we all know, walking in a confident and upbeat way tends to raise our spirits, as well as our shoulders.)

  - You might institute a circle dance to get people moving. Begin by moving your shoulders to a beat, and ask group members to join in. Then ask one person to show a dance move, and have the group follow. Go around a circle, so that all group members can demonstrate a move. To view a circle dance visit www.imnf.org/mhp-book-resources.

- Throughout this guidebook, there are many examples of rhythmic activities that involve synchronized movement between people with dementia and their caregivers. These activities have been shown to improve the mood and morale of caregivers, as well as patients. In other words, the effects are not specific to people with dementia. People with depression symptoms and emotional issues—*people in general!*—are likely to benefit from rhythmic activities that involve synchronized movement. See, for example, the closing exercise of a therapeutic drumming circle that includes people with dementia and staff experiencing many moments of human connection: www.imnf.org/mhp-book-resources. This exercise might work well in a music-based group that is focused on emotional wellness.

• See also the discussion of music interventions for people with Parkinson's disease (Module 7). There is a growing evidence base for the use of music therapy in the treatment of Parkinson's disease; and, ideally, people with Parkinson's are prescribed or offered many types of dance and exercise that address their special needs. Clinical experience shows that participation improves mood and morale, and helps some patients overcome depression symptoms that are often part of having Parkinson's. But here's the point: Many of these groups include family care partners and others who do not have Parkinson's disease—*and they benefit as well!* In fact, if you look at a Parkinson's dance group, you will not be able to tell who is a "patient" and who is not: the dance exercise appears to be an expressive and positive experience for both groups.

## TAKEAWAY

Music- and dance-based exercises that are prescribed for people with movement disorders may also be therapeutic for people with depression symptoms and other emotional issues. Review the video at www.imnf.org/mhp-book-resources. for ideas about what might work in your music-based group for people with depression symptoms or other emotional issues.

## Musical improvisation

In our examples so far we have seen that music therapists and other music partners may improvise new words to a familiar song, to reflect the interests and feelings of patients in the moment. **Music therapists are trained to improvise music as well as words; that is, they are able to make changes in the music, and even create new music, to respond to a person or a group in real time.**

**Improvisation is a basic tool of music therapy.** As our definition recognizes, music therapy takes place within a *therapeutic relationship* that is formed between a therapist and patient(s), through engagement with music. For this relationship to form, the music therapist must offer *the right music, at the right time.*

In much of this guidebook we focus on choosing the *right music* for an individual or group—for example, familiar songs with personal meaning, or songs that experience shows tend to be therapeutic for certain groups and clinical populations. With improvisation, we can go further; with improvisation, we can shape the music to what is needed in real time, in individual or group sessions.

Music therapists are trained to improvise around rhythm, melody, harmony, and other music components. This sounds complicated, and it is. If you are not a musician, you might find it challenging to improvise music at a moment's notice. But consider that you do something similar, *with your own voice*, all the time. Just as you might naturally lower your voice to calm a friend, or speak haltingly to gain their attention and convey your loving concern, so might a music therapist alter the pitch and rhythm of the music, to achieve similar effects.

## Why everyone can improvise—at some level

When we speak of improvisation, what often comes to mind are masterful improvisations performed by jazz artists. Or if you're a classical music devotee, you may think of composers like Mozart, who could produce gorgeous original melodies on the spot, for any occasion.

**But musical improvisation doesn't require that level of training or talent. Improvisation is something that everyone is able to do *at some level*.**

Most of us can improvise around musical rhythms and sounds; we express ourselves with movements, beating and tapping a drum, or with spontaneous vocalizations, sighing, humming, or singing. We've noted one example of this: during the Covid-19 pandemic, people were observed making music from their windows and balconies. They were improvising—making simple rhythms and expressive musical sounds, often with pots and pans. No musical training necessary.

Music is part of our culture—the sound culture that surrounds us from the moment of birth (and even before that). **Improvisation draws on our intuitive or unconscious understanding of the music with which we are familiar.** We will not all be talented composers, approaching the highest levels of musical expression—any more than we will all be literary stars, in speaking and writing our own language. But every one of us is able to improvise rhythms and sounds, as a form of communication. And that is important.

## Drawing on your experience

Although you may not realize it, you already have a strong grasp of the rules of music, and are primed to improvise rhythms and sounds that are meaningful to others. (You didn't have to be formally taught the basic rules of music, any more than you needed to be taught grammar in order to communicate a sentence!)

You can find evidence for this in your own experience. If you are listening to a child performing a simple piano piece that you have never heard before, you will likely recognize when a wrong note is played. The sound doesn't make sense, within the context of your expectations. You may also recognize when a rhythm has been violated. In particular, you have a strong sense of where the music is going, with respect to melody and harmony, at least with the music of your culture. If someone stops the music before a phrase is completed, your listening mind will likely fill in the missing tones.

In other words, you know more than you think you do. Music educator Joan Koenig notes that many parents are "terrified at the idea of improvising a musical activity because they believe that only talented musicians are capable of improvising even the most basic musical exchange" (Koenig, 2021, p.63). And caregivers may have the same reservations. But even three-year-olds are able to improvise when "playing" the piano. Koenig describes young children "caressing the keys" while singing, and notes that the words to the songs, like the music, are "deliciously approximate." She likens this to "musical scribbling." We all do it, if given the chance.

## Musical improvisation: A closer look

Typically, improvisations are led by music therapists or other music partners who serve as group leaders. Participants may enter into the musical dialogue in several ways. Here are some examples:

- Group members play a basic rhythm; the leader improvises a rhythmic variation in response or as accompaniment. The leader or a group member offers a rhythm or musical phrase, and other group members improvise their own "take" on this music. All group members will be able to improvise at some level; and for some, musical training and creativity will come into play.

- The leader invites a group member to sing, or play a solo on a rhythmic or melodic instrument, while being supported rhythmically by the group. For example, the soloist may sing, or play the xylophone or recorder, for a short interlude, while the group plays more softly, as background, until the signal is given (by the leader) for the soloist to rejoin the group.

- As follow-up, group discussion will focus on feelings, thoughts, and memories that have been elicited by the improvisation.

## Improvisation techniques and tips for group leaders
### Rhythmic improvisation: The basics
**As a first step, invite group members to imitate or echo a rhythm, sound, or melodic phrase.** As children, we learn to sing and make music by imitating; then improvising; and only sometimes by reading music notation. Children imitate adult music-makers by banging piano keys and singing along, sort of. You might begin your group by inviting members to imitate you, and one another, playing drums and rhythm instruments, and perhaps chanting.

- Offer group members drums, tambourines, and other rhythm instruments.

- Begin by playing a short rhythm (perhaps with chanted words) and ask members to *imitate* or echo your music. This has the advantage of first asking participants to do something they know they can do.

- After you have established the imitation, begin to improvise around your rhythm, one improvisation at a time; again, ask members to imitate or echo your music. This step will introduce members to the process of improvisation, and build their confidence.

- Next, ask each group member, in turn, to improvise their own "take" on a rhythm. Here is a chance for everyone to solo.

- Finally, or in a subsequent session, offer a simple rhythm and ask a group member to volunteer to lead an improvisation offering, say, four different improvisations on that rhythm. Group members will imitate and echo the improvisations.

  Alternatively, ask a group member to propose a rhythm, and play it several times for the group. Once the rhythm is established, go around the circle, asking each member to improvise their own take on the basic rhythm. These exercises encourage individual group members to take the lead in improvisations.

Note that group members may respond or "improvise" in many ways—moving to the music, humming or vocalizing, or listening actively to "catch" the emotional message conveyed by the improvisation.

### Adding improvisation around musical sounds

Music-based groups that improvise around rhythmic patterns can add pleasing musical sounds or tones to expand expressive possibilities. A variety of simple toned percussion instruments (played by striking with the hand or a drumstick) are available: these include tone bars, chime bars, wind chimes, resonator bars, and "harmony bars."

Each tonal instrument produces one or more musical sounds. Sets of tone bars are often based on five-tone (or pentatonic) musical scales that include only tones that are pleasing when played together—so it is impossible to make a "mistake" when improvising. When group members play these tones together, the result is a rich and harmonious sound environment, according to Remo, Inc., the music instrument manufacturer. Tonal percussion instruments are easy to play, and tend to inspire spontaneous improvisations among performers at all levels of musical experience, from young school children to seniors in a drumming circle or music-based group.

### Some benefits of improvisation

Improvisation tends to be therapeutic for people with depression symptoms. Here are some reasons why:

- Improvisation is an opportunity for self-expression.

- Participating in rhythmic improvisation tends to raise the energy level and interest of participants. Simply taking action, *speaking out in one's own rhythm*, can be therapeutic for people with depression symptoms.

- Brain science suggests that when a person is actively engaged in musical improvisation of any kind (for 15 minutes or more) some of the inhibitions that ordinarily restrict our movement and verbal functioning are not in play. This happens because the self-monitoring area of the brain "turns off" and the creative areas of the brain are fired up.

### Taking improvisation one step further: Improvising around familiar songs

Improvising songs and melodies requires moderate music improvisation skills. When carried out in a music-based group for therapeutic purposes, improvisation requires a leader with a background or training in music therapy concepts and interventions.

Here are some tips and strategies for group leaders with background or training in music therapy:

- As group leader, you can use improvisation to stimulate group discussion. After the group has played or listened to a musical selection, you will typically encourage members to verbalize their responses and explore associations with the music. **As you wait for verbal responses, try improvising on the music under discussion.** For example:

  - Softly repeat the melody or musical theme, slowly, as a kind of open-ended question.

  - Hum parts of the song as background, improvising as you seek responses.

  - **When gaps appear in discussion, improvise music that re-engages group members with the music.** For example, play the refrain (or other memorable passages) repeatedly, varying the dynamics; play the melody in a higher or lower octave, and so on. Strum a chord sequence that will "remind" group members of the emotional message of the song or music selection.

  - **Improvise in response to the discussion as it evolves.** When group members offer personal interpretations of a song, reflect that back to them in your playing or singing, if you are able. For example, suppose a group member says that a lively song makes her feel sad or nostalgic. You might improvise a version of the song that was slower, or in a minor key, to reflect her feelings—and ask others to respond to this variation. (This generally requires a moderate level of music improvisation skills.)

- Use the "Right Now!" improvisation to help group members open up. Ask a willing group member for a word that describes the moment, either emotionally or physically. Invite the group member to play a rhythmic or other instrument of their choice, and expand on the feeling of "right now." Invite other willing group members to do the same. Ask each member to describe the rhythmic or sound-making instrument, or the orchestral instrument, that might best communicate their emotional or physical state at this moment.

- After the group sings a familiar song, respond with a melodic improvisation. The melodic improvisation (or variation) might involve a simple change of dynamics, affecting how loud or soft different phrases are sung; changes in rhythm; changes in harmony, affecting the mood or texture of the song; the addition of decorative touches, such as trills, grace notes, turns, and glissandi (slides from one note to another), and so on. Improvisations can be simple or artful, depending on the musical training of the group leader.

- Improvise a simple passage of music—perhaps a series of "blues" chords, or a rock and roll rhythm with a simple melody. Ask group members, "What did that music feel like for you? What title would you give this musical composition?"

- Guide the group through an imaging or meditation exercise—for example, being on a beach at sunrise, and absorbing the rhythms of the ocean, wind, bird-life, and so on. Improvise music to accompany this experience as it evolves... Alternatively, create a beautiful ambience through music, a place of peace and wellness. Ask group members where they imagine this place is, and what it feels like. Let group members guide your music-making, through this happy place.

## Music-based groups for well seniors

There are some senior care communities that provide residents with life-enhancing amenities and activities that are not required by state regulations and are seldom reimbursed by Medicare/Medicaid or private insurance. Most important among these, we believe, are "creative aging" programs that promote lifetime learning and participation in high-quality creative arts activities. Through such programs, older people *at all levels of function* become students and student artists, as well as participants in community arts activities, performances, and audiences.

Music therapy and music-based programs play a key role in the creative aging environment. Today, in some full-service senior communities, music-based groups and activities may be offered to well seniors: for example, to seniors in assisted living who experience mild or occasional depression symptoms, to outpatients recovering well from recent hip surgery, and to well seniors in independent living situations that promise to support them in aging well. In this section, we will explore music-based groups for older people who are focused on wellness, and aging well.

### Wellness goals: What are they?

A general guide to music therapy goals, as related to social, emotional, cognitive, and motor skills, appears in Module 1. As you can see, some of these goals focus on mitigating or managing symptoms or conditions that are common among people in senior care settings. For example, goals such as "to improve awareness of self and others" or "to improve the ability to complete activities of daily care" are familiar treatment goals for people living with dementia. That said, most music therapy goals are appropriate for people at all levels of functioning—at one time or another. Who among us has not sought "to decrease stress and anxiety," or hoped "to achieve a heightened sense of awareness of self through proven accomplishments?" Who among us is not in search of opportunities "to experience exceptional moments of human interaction?"

## TAKEAWAY

Music-based groups for well seniors address many of the same goals that emerge in groups for people with health and mental health issues. This means that leaders of wellness groups can draw on the ideas and techniques that are presented throughout this guidebook. For example, the singing interventions that are described in Module 6 on dementia care may be adapted to the needs of wellness groups. By the same token, dance exercises that are described in Module 7, for people with Parkinson's disease, may help improve balance, prevent falls, and enhance the mood of well participants.

We should note that well seniors in assisted living situations may be referred to music-based groups by activities directors, who are not clinicians, but who are prepared to address the wellness needs of their residents. Seniors in independent living situations are often "self-referred," and likely to have formulated their own health or wellness goals.

Typically the health and wellness goals of well seniors are to:

- **maintain a current state of wellness.** This is often expressed as the need to avoid becoming sick or disabled, and dependent on others. (Not very upbeat—but nearly everyone says something to this effect at one time or another.)

- **cope, proactively, on an ongoing basis, with everyday "aches and pains," hearing/vision losses, and other common effects of aging.** In wellness terms, these goals energize people to make healthy lifestyle choices; to take action to prevent physical and emotional problems, especially cognitive decline; and remain active and independent.

Seniors who choose to participate in a music-based wellness group may have specific wellness goals, for example to "stay sharp" intellectually, or expand their social network (i.e. to prevent cognitive decline and social isolation).

- **adapt successfully to the mental health and spiritual challenges of the later years.** In wellness terms, this means to age and evolve in a way that enables one to live fully, coping with inevitable losses, and retaining a capacity for enjoyment and engagement with life. In general, a person's way of responding to the challenges of aging reflects their way of coping with earlier life events. The music-based wellness group is an opportunity for members to revisit and share life events, through music, memories, and discussion. It's also an opportunity for participants to share coping strategies that have been successful, or mostly so, in common life situations.

- **grow and develop.** An outstanding feature of successful adaptation is that it leaves the way open for future growth (Vaillant, 1977). **For well seniors, clinical music therapy goals can be framed as opportunities for growth and development.** For example, "To increase social interactions" might include "to remain open to new intimate and social relationships"—for example, to become a mentor (or mentee?) making music with young rap artists in the community, or to imagine the possibility of falling in love and marrying in one's eighties. Goals for self-expression might be realized through music interventions in the group, and also through group members' participation in creative aging programs that provide arts education and experiences in a variety of disciplines. (See "A creative aging approach" in Module 3.)

Group leaders will begin by acknowledging the expressed needs of well seniors who opt into wellness groups; and they will need to select music and frame group discussions accordingly. This should not be difficult, because the needs of older people, to grow and develop (even in adversity), are widely shared. Which is to say they are our needs, too.

## Suggestions for leaders of music-based groups for well seniors

Here are some framings that may work for your group:

- Begin the session by playing familiar music as background, and proceed to go around the group asking members to introduce themselves and share their wellness goals. How do they pursue these goals, or hope to pursue them? Wellness is about making healthy choices, around exercise and physical activity, diet, stress, and mood management, for example. Ask participants what enters into their choices.

Specifically, how does music (listening to music, singing or playing a rhythmic or melodic instrument) support their self-described wellness goals? Discussion prompts might focus on stress management, motivation for exercise or physical activity, opportunities for learning new skills, and so on. What do members hope to achieve through participation in a music-based wellness group?

- As noted, a primary goal of many older people is to maintain cognitive health—to "stay sharp," avoid memory lapses now and memory impairment later. Ask group members how they address this goal; what do they think they need to do to maintain brain health? Perhaps they focus on activities such as doing crossword puzzles and Sudoku, attending lectures and discussion groups, and so forth. (In the absence of evidence, avoid commenting on the effectiveness of these activities.) Open up the discussion to include other activities group members enjoy that might contribute to cognitive health. Begin by suggesting exercise and physical activities—including (especially) moving to music.

  Numerous studies show that physical activity improves brain health; on the other hand, physical inactivity has been shown to be the most significant risk factor in cognitive decline, and the development of dementia (Barnes & Yaffe, 2011, as cited in Gupta, 2021). Dance interventions have been shown to support cognitive health for older people: learning and remembering dance steps, as in ballroom dancing, is a cognitive task. To date, one major study of the effect of leisure activities on the risk of dementia in older people found that dancing was the only activity associated with lower risk of dementia (Verghase et al., 2003). In addition, of course, dance and physical exercise provide many other health benefits, and often pleasure.

## TAKEAWAY

Group leaders can draw on the moving to music interventions described in this module, and throughout this guidebook, to help group members meet their goals for brain health wellness.

- **Music-making also has the potential to build and maintain brain health.** Learning new musical skills is intellectually stimulating at any age, "because music is a complex medium that allows for growth and development and demands some intellectual activity in order to maintain an acquired competency level" (Clair, 1996, p.43).

## TAKEAWAY

Leaders of wellness groups can draw on music-making, singing, and rhythmic and sound improvisations, described throughout this guidebook, to help group members meet their needs for brain health, as well as the physical and emotional strengths that support independence and other wellness goals.

- **Music engagement can also help older people manage pain, including common aches and pains**, and the experience of chronic pain. Using music while exercising, for example, helps people of all ages press themselves beyond their usual limits (which is what older people often find themselves determined to do). That's because music that is pleasing to us drives the release of neurotransmitters in the brain that reduce the intensity of pain, in part by dampening the pain signal.

  The analgesic or painkiller effect is physiological, because the pain signal is reduced, and also psychological, because a better emotional state is established, and that helps diminish the stress related to pain.

  Personal responses to pain vary widely; but most people find that music that captures their attention will distract them from pain and discomfort, or at least lower the intensity of the pain experience. And for people with chronic pain, music may have the potential to be developed as a non-pharmacological self-management treatment.

## TAKEAWAY

Leaders of wellness groups can help participants explore ways in which listening and moving to pleasurable music will help manage occasional or chronic pain. Consultation with a music therapist can also provide protocols for coping with chronic pain through music therapy, as part of a healthcare plan for those who are motivated to pursue this path to wellness.

- Music engagement has become a well-accepted (and evidence-based) wellness strategy for older people who are the primary consumers of healthcare in the US, and everywhere. The National Institute on Aging of the NIH has looked at the research and announced that "Participating in the arts creates paths to healthy aging" (2019). NIA points out that "we all know to eat right, exercise, and get a good night's sleep to stay healthy. But can flexing our creative muscles help us thrive as we age?" The answer is yes—and leaders of wellness groups can expand on that, as they engage participants in music interventions and discussion.

# MODULE 5

# Music for People Living with Dementia

Family caregivers, professional caregivers, CNAs, HHAs—everyone who is involved in caring for a person with dementia—need to ask themselves: Can you imagine a dementia that includes joy—even momentary joy—for you, for your family member, or the patients you care for? *Can you imagine that?*

Tia Powell, MD, is a professor of psychiatry and bioethics, and part of a family that has been affected by dementia. Powell wants to find a way to build a life of joy and dignity for people with dementia, and for all of us, "from beginning to end." Her book *Dementia Reimagined* views dementia through the lenses of history, modern medicine, and personal memoir. The book is a full-hearted resource for our time—and music is only one part of it. But it is significant that Powell begins *Dementia Reimagined* by telling us about an evening she spent in Manhattan at a concert by The Unforgettables, a chorus made up of people with dementia and their caregivers. It was, as Powell describes it, a beautiful experience, that left people dancing in the aisles, literally, "with delight and dignity"—and with many, herself included, "with eyes misting over."

Powell writes:

> Here's a way…to help you imagine a dementia that contains joy. The capacity to enjoy and respond to music outlasts many other cognitive functions; even after spontaneous speech has become difficult, many people can still sing lyrics to songs learned long ago. Even in advanced disease when happiness is hard to come by, people can respond to music they love. (Powell, 2019, p.11)

This is a powerful idea, but not a new idea. More than 40 years ago, we began to observe and explore the effects of music therapy on people with dementia in a nursing home. Clinical experience and emerging brain research have provided evidence for the use of music-based therapies to help people with dementia, at all stages of the disease.

## What is dementia?

Dementia is a *syndrome* characterized by a progressive decline in memory and other mental abilities, almost always in older people. A "syndrome," in medicine, is a *group of symptoms* that occur together (possibly in different combinations), and which define, or at least help us diagnose, a disease such as dementia.

In dementia, the symptoms show up as problems in remembering, learning, planning, paying attention, and completing a task at hand. Over time, people with dementia lose the memory and mental abilities that are necessary to perform in their usual capacities, at work and at home. Eventually, they are unable to manage activities of daily living, such as dressing, bathing, and toileting. Language may become impoverished or impaired, as the person increasingly struggles to find words. Without the grounding of shared memories, communication with others becomes difficult, and less frequent. These losses, in turn, may create agitation, anxiety, and depression. The way and degree to which symptoms are expressed varies from person to person.

Dementia is a "neurocognitive disorder"—in other words, a brain disorder. It is thought to be caused by a loss of function or structure of neurons in the brain. But it affects the whole person, not just cognition, but also personality and behavior—potentially, everything.

People who are diagnosed with dementia in its early stages live on average for about ten years; but this depends on the severity of the disease on diagnosis, and on many other factors; and it is not unusual for people to live with dementia for as many as 20 years. The disease is *progressive* (meaning it gets worse over time), *irreversible*, and, in time, fatal. But we are talking about a lot of time in the lives of our patients; and we know that these lives have meaning—the same way our lives do. So what we want to do, as caregivers, is find ways to care for people with dementia that recognize the meaning in their lives, and support their pursuit of happiness, in the circumstances in which they find themselves.

## What do we mean by "Alzheimer's and related dementias?"

Not long ago, people with dementia went without any firm diagnosis. This is because dementia is not one specific disease. It is a syndrome or group of symptoms that are characteristic of a number of diseases that we have come to call "dementia." The reference that physicians use for diagnosis of mental disorders, the *Diagnostic and Statistical Manual of Mental Disorders, fifth edition* (DSM-5) (American Psychiatric Association, 2022), has named dementia a "neurocognitive disorder."

Today, a person with dementia is likely to be diagnosed with Alzheimer's disease. In fact, Alzheimer's disease accounts for between 60 and 80 percent of all cases, depending on your source. Alzheimer's has a high public profile (it's well branded!). The Alzheimer's Association is a powerful national presence, providing information, support groups, and advocacy for people with Alzheimer's and related dementias and their caregivers.

In 2021, more than six million Americans age 65 and older are living with Alzheimer's. Most (72%) are age 75 or older, and almost two-thirds are women. Older Black Americans are about twice as likely as older White Americans to have Alzheimer's or related dementias; older Hispanic Americans are about one and half times as likely to be affected. The populations of long-term memory care programs in the US tend to reflect these demographics. The majority of people with Alzheimer's and related dementias live in the community, cared for by family members and unpaid (non-professional) caregivers. Even so, people with dementia make up a large proportion of older Americans in adult day services or nursing home care (Alzheimer's Association, n.d.).

## Types of dementia

Although Alzheimer's disease is the most common and best-known type of dementia, there are other forms of dementia, with different contributing causes, and variations in the symptoms experienced. If you want to learn more about types of dementia, you can use the same reference that physicians use, the *DSM-5-TR Neurocognitive Disorders Supplement*, October 2022, available here at www.imnf.org/mhp-book-resources.

To use music therapeutically with people with dementia, it is usually not necessary to know the specific type of dementia that has been diagnosed. However, there is an important exception: people with frontotemporal dementia (FTD) experience changes in the part of the brain that affects their ability to hear musical tones, which may be perceived as noise. This, and changes in behavior and personality, are generally contraindications for therapeutic music activities for people with this form of dementia.

It is important to note that dementia—or apparent symptoms of dementia—may be observed in connection with other medical conditions that affect people in senior care settings. For example, dementias are part of the symptomology of Parkinson's disease and Huntington's disease. In addition, dementia at varying levels of severity may be associated with traumatic brain injury (TBI), multiple sclerosis, HIV/AIDS, or even malnutrition (such as a lack of thiamine or vitamin B1).

Dementia symptoms may also be induced or brought about by substance or drug (ab)use, or by medications that interfere with cognitive functions. Medications commonly given to older people, for everything from urinary incontinence to depression, may have side effects that mimic dementia. These side effects include memory and attention problems, agitation and confusion, "mental slowing" reflected in communication and social responses, and other symptoms.

## Stages of dementia

Dementia develops gradually, in stages. Mild to moderate dementia often lasts for years; and during this time, people with dementia are able to enjoy many of the things they enjoyed in the past, including the company of family and friends, and manageable activities that give pleasure and purpose. Most people with mild or moderate symptoms live at home, with support from family members.

**People with dementia who are living in long-term or memory care settings are most likely to have moderate to severe symptoms, and to require help with activities of daily living. They too may be able to enjoy activities that give pleasure and purpose to life, including participation in social activities and religious services, music listening and music-making, exercise, gardening, and other activities well adapted to their interests and capabilities. Even in the late stage of dementia, a person may respond to rhythmic activities, familiar songs, a familiar voice, a human touch (as in a hand massage), and possibly other stimuli.**

Across the stages of dementia, the experiences of patients differ, reflecting the uniqueness of each person. Some patients show a rapid deterioration of cognitive function, whereas with others, cognitive declines are much slower. In some people, the onset of dementia seems to accentuate certain personality traits that have been well controlled in the past. (For example, an opinionated or self-dramatizing person may become more so—the same lovable and eccentric uncle at the holiday table, but now out of control and less responsive to the environment.) In other people, the uniqueness of the personality seems to be lost (Takeda *et al.*, 2012, as cited in Gentner, 2017). Among people with dementia, skills deteriorate at surprisingly different rates: "Some simple aptitudes such as the ability to remember a few objects may be long gone before seemingly higher-level ones, such as singing a song, begin to decline" (Benveniste *et al.*, 2014, p.4, as cited in Gentner, 2017).

## TAKEAWAY

Each person with dementia is on their own personal journey. And yet dementia has a course of its own, as we all know. Descriptions of the stages of dementia have been developed by healthcare professionals and caregivers to help them meet the needs of people with dementia, in the moment and as the disease progresses. Figure 3 shows one example.

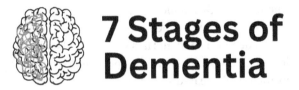

# 7 Stages of Dementia

| Stage 1 | No Dementia | No Cognitive Decline | - Normal function<br>- No memory loss<br>- People with NO dementia and no subjective or objective cognitive decline are considered in Stage 1 |
| --- | --- | --- | --- |
| Stage 2 | No Dementia | Very Mild Cognitive Decline | - Complains of memory deficits such as names they normally recall well<br>- Symptoms not evident to loved ones or doctors |
| Stage 3 | No Dementia | Mild Cognitive Decline | - Increased forgetfulness<br>- Slight difficulty concentrating<br>- Decreased work performance in demanding settings<br>- May misplace an object of value<br>- Difficulty finding right words and names<br>- Loved ones begin to notice |
| Stage 4 | Early-Stage | Moderate Cognitive Decline | - Difficulty concentrating<br>- Forgets recent events<br>- Difficulties managing finances<br>- Difficulties with traveling alone to new places<br>- Difficulty completing tasks<br>- In denial about symptoms<br>- Socialization problems: Withdraws from friends or family<br>- Cognitive problems can be detected with a careful evaluation |
| Stage 5 | Mid-Stage | Moderately Severe Cognitive Decline | - Major memory deficiencies<br>- Needs assistance with choosing the proper clothing to wear<br>- May not know their correct address or phone number<br>- May not know the date or season or the day of the week |
| Stage 6 | Mid-Stage | Severe Cognitive Decline | - Cannot carry out ADLs without help<br>- Forgets names of close family members such as their spouse<br>- Forgets recent events<br>- Forgets major events in past<br>- Difficulty counting down from 10<br>- Incontinence (loss of bladder and subsequently bowel control)<br>- Progressive difficulty speaking<br>- Personality and emotional changes<br>- Delusions, e.g., accusing spouse of being someone else<br>- Anxiety and agitation |
| Stage 7 | Late-Stage | Very Severe Cognitive Decline (Late Dementia) | - Cannot speak or communicate meaningfully<br>- Requires help with most activities<br>- Progressive loss of motor skills such as ability to walk, sit up, smile and hold their head up |

*Figure 3: Seven stages of dementia (source: Dementia Care Central, www.dementiacarecentral.com/aboutdementia/facts/stages)*

## Music to meet the social and emotional needs of people with dementia

Dementia (as a "neurocognitive disorder") has the most significant effect on cognition or thinking: in the public imagination, the loss of memory is the defining characteristic of dementia. But anyone who has lived with or cared for a person with dementia knows that this disease affects social emotional life as well. Dementia is, in fact, a mental illness, with all that implies—the emotional distress and problematic behavior.

If you work with dementia patients in a senior care facility, you will find that most patients exhibit problems in the social and emotional domains. These problems include decreased self-awareness, withdrawal, depression, agitation, confusion, anger, and despair.

**Social and emotional problems are partly due to the nature of dementia (that is, brain damage), but the environment also plays a role. When a person experiencing memory loss is admitted to senior care, the unfamiliar environment may cause confusion, fear, or fear-motivated aggression. Memory loss, and an environment of strangers, can easily lead to social withdrawal.**

We can support people living with dementia, by providing person-centered care, in a setting that includes fulfilling activities, a welcoming social and physical environment—*and music!* Music is a powerful therapeutic tool, enhancing person-centered care, and helping patients and caregivers find, together, "a dementia that contains joy."

### Familiar songs

In the late 1970s, a few of us who worked in nursing homes began to notice that music can have "an almost magical power" on patients:

> In Alzheimer's disease...you can have patients who are unable to talk, unable to organize themselves, patients who are agitated and confused. Music for them can have an almost magical power by eliciting memories and associations and restoring to them moods, the memories, the fluency, and the feeling of their former selves and their former lives. (Sacks, 1991)

The music that had the almost magical effect was not just any music. It was music that was familiar and meaningful to the patients with dementia: songs their mother sang to them at bedtime; songs that were popular when they fell in love and married; or perhaps songs that were part of the community, a traditional holiday song or church hymn. The music had the potential to restore to these patients the feeling of their former lives *because it came from their former lives.*

But familiar songs don't work by themselves.

To have a real effect, familiar songs should be heard or sung in partnership with a music therapist or someone else who is trained to engage with the patient through music. The music partner may be a CNA, HHA, or a family care partner.

A familiar song may elicit memories and associated feelings, yet these memories and associations may be, for our patient, fragmented, wordless, even formless in ordinary terms. The music therapist or other music partner can support the memory work, by encouraging the person with dementia to express the memory and associations that are prompted by the music. This helps the person access the memory—and the feeling of their former self—at that moment.

The moment is special. And when these moments happen on a regular basis, there's a chance that the person with dementia will become more alert each time, and recognition will extend over longer periods. For example, a patient who was seen at the IMNF had not recognized his wife for a few years. We began to work with him using familiar songs. After participating in an hour-long group program three times a week for three months, he was able to recognize his wife when she came to visit. He called her by name and asked her where she had been all this time!

**How to use familiar songs in dementia care**
There are two ways for music therapists and others to use familiar songs in a care setting:

- By singing and playing live music:

  *Examples:*

  A recreation therapist sings and plays familiar songs with members of a dementia group.

  A family care partner sings a song, as she seeks to involve her mom in preparing dinner. (It's a song from her childhood, one her mother used to sing to her.)

  A HHA sings a song that her patient seems to like as she prepares her medications.

- By using pre-recorded music:

  *Examples:*

  A music therapist and CNA make a personalized playlist of a person's favorite songs and puts it on an iPod, iPhone, or MP3 player. The CNA then facilitates the use of the playlist, and monitors the listening sessions to ensure a positive experience. (See the section on personalized playlists later in this module.)

A family care partner or HHA uses a personalized playlist, or provides other access to the favorite music of the person with dementia, to engage the person during care activities.

### The music-based dementia group: Singing and playing and listening to familiar songs

Music therapists and other music partners often present familiar songs in a group setting: that is, they function as group leaders. Often group leaders sing and play the songs themselves. But it also works for the leader to deliver familiar songs from pre-recorded sources, reaching out to the group the same way a singer does.

Here are some pointers to help you get started as a group leader for a dementia group:

- **Begin by creating a safe space of caring and acknowledging each individual. Through engagement with the music, you can create *a therapeutic relationship* with individual group members, if only in the moment.**

   Shared music experiences have a way of creating a sense of togetherness that works, even if words are not exchanged. In the moment, the person is *attuned, in time, in harmony*, with another person or persons, through the music. For people living with dementia, hearing their favorite music in the company of someone who is interacting and holding their attention creates a safe space and enhances their experience in the moment. Often, with repetition, these moments of connection are reached more and more easily—a desirable outcome.

- It's an advantage if you are able to sing simple songs, closely approximating accurate pitch, rhythm, and phrasing. Many people can do this; musical training is not necessary. Listening to a song (for example, on YouTube) and singing along is good practice for those who feel they need it.

- If you do not feel confident singing, you can use pre-recorded songs from internet sources, such as YouTube or Spotify. But do not sit back and listen to the song, passively. Try to help *deliver* the song, as a singer would, with expressive gestures and facial expressions. Or be actively present, sharing the song and the experience delivered by memorable artists, such as Frank Sinatra or Elvis Presley.

- Music therapists and recreation therapists often accompany themselves, usually on guitar or keyboard. Rhythm instruments, such as drums or tambourines, also may be used by the music partner (and may also be distributed to group members). CNAs, HHAs, musician volunteers, and other music partners can often provide guitar or keyboard accompaniment for well-known songs—but this is not necessary. The voice, alone, is a powerful instrument.

  An option for music partners is to sing with a recorded backup—but only if this can be done easily, without technical difficulties or interruptions.

- **Face-to-face contact—including eye contact—is extremely important in making a connection and helping patients remain alert.** When using recorded music as accompaniment, or in place of live music, avoid performance tasks that require fiddling with technology settings. And, as always, make sure the equipment is charged and ready, and working well.

## Choosing familiar songs

The first step in using familiar songs is, of course, to identify those songs that are "familiar" to the person with dementia; and if you are working with a group, you will need to identify songs that everyone will know.

1. The age of your patients is your best guide to what songs are likely to be "familiar" as well as personally meaningful. Research shows that people tend to remember—and respond to—songs that were popular when they were teenagers and young adults; these songs are somehow encoded, in the brain, along with the emotionally charged events of these years, to make us who we are. In general, slowish songs, with sentimental, loving, or inspirational messages, are at the top of the "familiar song" list, and easiest to use. If your patients are in their eighties and nineties, try "You Are My Sunshine" or "As Time Goes By" or "My Funny Valentine." Song lists for different age groups have been developed by music therapists to help you identify songs that are likely familiar and meaningful to your patients. Visit www.imnf.org/mhp-book-resources to access song lists for various age groups.

2. Especially for a group, choose songs that seem to relate to shared experiences. For example, try songs like "White Christmas" or "Take Me Out to the Ball Game." Also effective are songs that we sing to children, such as "Yankee Doodle," and songs that are well loved as part of a shared culture, such as "Somewhere Over the Rainbow."

3. **Give careful attention, as always, to the cultural or ethnic backgrounds of the patients with whom you are working.** Songs from the "old country," traditional songs in a given sub-culture, or hymns sung in religious settings are good possibilities. Song lists for people of different cultures and ethnic backgrounds in the US have been compiled by music therapists to help you meet the needs of your patients. Visit www.imnf.org/mhp-book-resources to access song lists for diverse ethnic groups in the US.

4. Music therapists have developed ways to identify songs that have deep personal meaning for individual patients. This involves a special kind of history-taking, ideally based on interviews with both the patient and family members. The personalized approach, as reflected in the personalized playlist, expands the options for therapy. In some cases, knowing the best-loved songs from a person's early years is the key to reaching that person even in the late stage of dementia. (See section on personalized playlists later in this module.)

## Establishing a secure and welcoming environment

It is crucial that the group leader maintains a closely attentive presence throughout the entirety of the group session. Here are some ways to establish a secure environment:

- Provide immediate and clear assurance and encouragement, such as nodding, tapping on knees, or using exaggerated vocal, facial, and bodily mirroring. These are behaviors that we tend to use naturally, and joyfully, with young children, because they are easily understood, without words. They have a place here.

- Maintain face-to-face and eye contact throughout the session.

- **Project a sense of personal stability and confidence.** The group leader should be seen as someone who can use music to respond to patients' emotions and help center them, safely, in the session.

- **Provide a consistent yet flexible session structure, over time.** Members of your group will welcome consistency, and a familiar routine, as well as new songs, and new challenges. Some group leaders like to start every session with a "hello" or greeting song, and close with a "goodbye" or closure song, in order to create a sense of security.

## What to expect

With the use of familiar songs you will usually see:

- more relaxed facial expressions, and less observable tension among group members

- a reduction in evident emotional distress, including frustration and confusion in group members; an immediate cessation of disruptive vocalizations and repetitive complaints

- spontaneous engagement in the music, including emotional engagement (a huge advance!)

- increased motivation towards self-expression and interaction with others, both verbal and nonverbal.

You may also see other responses that tell you that your patients are engaged in the music experience, with positive results. These include:

- barely detectable finger- or foot-tapping to a song's rhythm among group members who may have been unresponsive and withdrawn

- spontaneous yet nearly inaudible singing of the lyrics

- subtle changes in affect, meaning the feelings that are expressed or can be observed: for example, less worry, more empathy or care for others

- a sudden request for repeating a song from a person who was previously uninterested or unresponsive.

## Familiar songs: A thought experiment

Imagine that you are in a car, alone, at night, speeding along a highway with spotty lighting, and no signs. It should not be a problem—you've been this way before. People are waiting for you, people you love. And yet you don't know where you are, or where you are going. Your GPS is working, but sometimes not; or maybe you haven't put in the right information (it's hard to tell). And every so often, someone you did not see comes speeding by... Your phone (where's my phone?) tells you the time, but nothing else.

Maybe they aren't even waiting for you anymore?!

You turn on your car radio. It is set to your favorite station. It plays a song you used to know—you tell yourself, yeah man, I used to dance to that song, with Her. You hold the wheel, as you used to hold Her, feeling the rhythm. You tap the wheel. She's not here now. You remember that. You'll talk about it later...because they are waiting for you. Yeah. You breathe easier. You know this road.

(BUT: What if you were in a rental car? And you turned on the radio and got a local news station, taking call-ins in a town you did not know? Or a station playing that loud electronic kind of music—what do they call it? Or songs announced and sung in some other language?)

> **TAKEAWAY**
> A person with moderate dementia may become dislocated and scared, even in what should be familiar circumstances. Familiar songs, which have personal meaning, provide context, memories, reminders of who and where we are, even when we are lost, in dementia or otherwise. The music is not only heard, but also felt in the body. In this case, moving to the rhythm of the song diffuses the anxiety of the person in the car, and this allows him to think more clearly.

## Live music in the day room

In skilled nursing facilities and other long-term facilities, there are often whole floors of residents with dementia and other disabilities that significantly limit their opportunities for social and sensory stimulation. These residents are nearly always in wheelchairs, if only to prevent falls and unattended wandering. They tend to be assembled in the day room or smaller common areas on the floor. The television is always on. There is little social interaction, unless organized by staff.

Ideally, residents with dementia and others in long-term care would be offered music-based groups of the kind we have described. But in institutions without a music therapy program or staff training, there's another option: live music can be provided on the floors and day rooms by per diem music therapists, recreation therapists, and musician volunteers. The music presenter will rely on medleys of familiar songs, always choosing those that have the greatest chance of emotionally engaging the residents on that floor.

For example, a musician volunteer, who has received some training in medical settings, will wheel a keyboard onto the floor, approaching patients in wheelchairs in the hallways and day room. (A guitar or accordion works as well.) The goal is a therapeutic experience—not entertainment. Here are some tips for providing live music for residents on the floor, in long-term settings:

- The musician volunteer on the floor uses many of the strategies of a successful group leader—acknowledging and greeting patients by name, looking each person in the eyes, even touching a patient lightly on the arm, in the manner of a family visitor. The difference is that the patients are not in a group, and may not be aware of one another. So the musician tends to relate to each person, one by one, in turn—almost like a strolling violinist in a café, going from one table to another.

- The musician will choose songs that resonate with each person. He will look for evidence of engagement—feet moving, fingers strumming on the table, lips moving to the music. In the day room, the musician may encounter one or two patients who are alert and eager to sing along. Others will need to be awakened, and encouraged. It helps to call out individuals by name ("Hey Esther, you're singing... Come on Jose, help me out!").

- Choosing a familiar song with a resonant refrain is one way of getting the group to come together.

*Example:*

As an example, picture this: The musician volunteer chooses the song "I'll be Loving You, Always." (The lyrics can be found on the internet.) He sings the lyrics moving from resident to resident, looking each in the eyes as he leans in on the word "always." He uses a passionate voice.

> I'll be loving you *always*
> With a love that's true *always*.
> When the things you've planned
> Need a helping hand,
> I will understand *always*.
>
> Always.
>
> Days may not be fair *always*,
> That's when I'll be there *always*.
> Not for just an hour,
> Not for just a day,
> Not for just a year,
> But *always*.

One by one, the group members chime in on "always." The song, as presented, transforms them from isolated individuals to a group in which each person is recognized and loved, not just for this moment, but "always" (based on an observation of D.F. Jarvis, May 11, 2022, at Wartburg).

## TAKEAWAY

Live music on the floor or day room can be therapeutic if presented by a music therapist or a musician volunteer who understands, even intuitively, the basics of music therapy (and the power of familiar songs).

## Using pre-recorded music: Personalized playlists

iPod listening programs, with personalized playlists, are a relatively inexpensive way of delivering familiar songs to people with dementia, and using this technology requires only minimal staff training. Here's how it works:

- A music therapist, recreation therapist, CNA, or HHA makes up a personalized playlist of a person's favorite songs and records them on an iPod, iPhone, or MP3 player. The playlist is unique to the individual and autobiographical (meaning it is based on their life experiences). Input from the patient and family helps inform the selection process.

- As a first step, the CNA or other frontline caregiver listens to the full playlist with the patient to ensure that none of the selections has an adverse effect on the patient (and that there are no technical difficulties). Adverse or negative effects sometimes occur for reasons that can't be anticipated: perhaps the playlist was created with input from a relative who has misjudged the likely effect of a song from the past, or perhaps the patient, at this time of life, has become vulnerable to emotional distress over memories associated with a favorite song. **The personalized playlist *must be reviewed* to ensure that the listening experience has the potential to be therapeutic for the patient.**

- The CNA, HHA, or family care partner facilitates the use of the playlist, helping the patient use the equipment, headphones, and so on, and arranging for the listening session to occur at an appropriate time, and in a quiet, comfortable setting.

- In long-term care, ideally the CNA will listen along with the patient in the course of everyday care—but this is not always possible. In any case, the CNA or a staff member remains present, or within reach, during the listening session, and makes descriptive notes (or a record), capturing observable changes in the patient's behavior or mood. The CNA engages with the patient, and helps give form to memories that emerge from the listening experience.

## Henry, "Alive Inside"

iPod listening programs, with personalized playlists, came to public attention in 2011, when an organization named Music & Memory posted a video of "Henry," a person living with dementia in a nursing home, who had barely said a word to anyone for years. Music & Memory had set up an iPod program in the nursing home, and Henry was given an iPod with his personal playlist. In the video, we see Henry come alive he listens to the songs on his iPod. And something comes alive in us as we experience this with him. The video has been viewed by more than seven million people to date.

Watch "Alive Inside" at www.imnf.org/mhp-book-resources.

Note that as you watch Henry it's not just the iPod, or the music, that effects this transformation.

Members of the healthcare team, and Henry's family, interact with him through the music. Henry communicates his feelings and memories to others in his environment. (And through the genius of the filmmaker, he communicates with us too.)

Everything about this is intentional, and based on what music therapists have learned about the therapeutic use of music with people with dementia. A personal playlist has been created for Henry from the music he loves. Staff have been made aware of Henry's history with music: "He was always singing," his daughter tells them; "every occasion he would come out with a song." The nursing home—the healthcare team—is supportive, and ready to learn about the power of music.

Below is a music assessment questionnaire developed by Music & Memory, the organization that pioneered, and continues to promote, the use of personalized playlist programs for people like Henry, in senior care settings. You can use the form to develop a personalized playlist for your patients. (A downloadable HANDOUT is available at www.imnf.org/mhp-book-resources.)

# MUSIC ASSESSMENT QUESTIONNAIRE

Listener's name: _____

Age: _____

Date: _____

Where did you grow up? _____

First language: _____

Do you have a favorite type of music? (Be as specific as possible.)

_____

What music did you listen to when you were young?

_____

Who was your favorite singer, group, band, orchestra?

_____

Did you sing at church/religious services?

_____

What religion/denomination, and what part of the country?

_____

Favorite hymns or other religious music?

_____

Did you enjoy going to Broadway shows or musicals?

_____

Did you have favorite TV shows or movies? (Theme songs from shows or movie soundtracks can elicit responses.)

_____

Do you remember going to see live music (rock, symphony, ballet, jazz, polka, clubs)?

_____

Do you like to dance?

_____

What type of dance?

_____

Do you have a favorite classical music composer (or composers)?

_____

What songs did you dance to at your wedding (or family weddings)?

_____

Were you in the armed services? If so, what branch, years, and where did you serve?

_____

Do you still have any records, tapes, and CDs that were favorites?

_____

Where can I find them?

_____

Can you hum any favorite songs? (You can use Shazam to identify the song if you don't know it.)

_____

Other notes:

_____

_____

_____

_____

_____

_____

NOTE: Music & Memory also provides guidance for song selection for nonverbal participants in a playlist program (see "How to be a Music Detective" at www.imnf.org/mhp-book-resources).

Today there are iPod personalized listening programs available in many senior care settings that serve dementia patients; and organizations like AARP promote these programs to family caregivers.

## Music for relaxation

Relaxation techniques using familiar music are effective in reducing physical and emotional tension in people with dementia.

- The music therapist, or music partner, must be keenly attuned to patients' physical and emotional states, in order to guide them carefully and gradually through the relaxation process. In working with a group, you might may begin with soft music, either recorded or performed on a guitar or other acoustic instrument, to set a relaxed mood. While gauging the responses of participants, the music therapist will move close to those individuals who need more direct attention and support.

- **Soft and steady drumbeats often set patients' physical and emotional states into a relaxed mode. Make sure that the drumbeats are steady, in the rhythm you establish. It is recommended that the tempo begins by matching the human heart beat, at 65 BPM (beats per minute), then gradually becomes slower.**

- Using your voice to match a patient's mood is effecting in reassuring patients and helping them feel safe. Your voice should be soft and steady, with pauses between the words, as needed, to create a calm and lolling rhythm.

## Music to enhance cognition

Cognition refers broadly to all the ways we think, learn, and remember. Included are high-order mental or "intellectual" skills, such as reasoning, planning, and problem-solving. Also included are abilities that don't seem to relate to "thinking" as we usually define it.

Cognition includes *perception*. The brain processes information—that's what it does. And all of our cognitive functions depend on how we perceive and organize this information, as it comes to us, moment by moment, through our sensory organs (eyes, ears, skin, etc.), and through our bodily sense of ourselves.

## Cognitive impairment in dementia

Perception develops in the first months of life, and auditory perception in the months before birth. As we begin to explore our environment, we develop expectations as to what will happen if, for example, we touch or strike something (a drum?), or if we hear a certain voice talking or singing. We don't "think" about what will happen, at 18 months of age, when we strike a drum; but the brain already knows what will happen. This is evidence of what we call "cognition."

Cognition also makes possible our use of symbols, including words and gestures. The developing child masters simple words, then language, and the infinite possibilities of thought and expression that language makes possible.

All of cognition is at risk in dementia. In the early stages of dementia, a person typically has difficulties with higher-order functions, such as planning events, learning new phone or computer skills, or just concentrating on tasks at hand. In the late stages of dementia, a person loses the ability to use or respond to words and gestures in a meaningful way. But, even then, the basic level of cognition involved in responding to sounds and feelings is retained. If a person in the later stages of dementia touches a drum, and makes a sound, they may do this again to produce that sound. If a person with dementia hears a voice, singing, it may have an effect—on memory, on expectation and mood—even though the person may not "know" who is singing, or what the song "means."

In long-term and memory care settings, caregivers must typically address a full range of cognitive impairments in dementia patients.

## Music for alertness and attention

For people with dementia, impairments in cognitive function may include the memory losses that we easily notice, as well as problems in perception, including decreased alertness and attention span, unintelligible language, and disturbances of thought around self-identity. If a person is not alert or attentive, they won't be able to respond, or learn something new—such as new daily care regimens, or the names of new people in their environment. If a person doesn't have a sense of their own identity, at a given moment, they may become seriously disoriented and unable to communicate in a way that is understood.

Familiar songs are very helpful in communicating with patients, as these songs so often give patients access to memories, with positive cognitive and emotional effects. But familiar songs—especially if presented in group, week after week—become very familiar indeed. And as we all know, it is something unexpected that gets and holds our attention.

Here are some ways to enhance alertness and attention:

- Leave out words of familiar lyrics while singing to prompt word retrieval. For example, "You are my...(sunshine), my only...(sunshine); You make me...(happy) when skies are...(gray)."

- Use a "passionate voice" to increase attention, along with other facial and/or hand cues, such as touching or tapping on limbs.

- Play or sing new songs that are likely to be "culturally familiar" to the group, though perhaps not familiar to every group member. This may facilitate a process of "recognizing" and "recalling."

- Manipulate the changes in the energy and direction of music dynamics (loudness vs. softness) to help patients stay alert and attentive.

- **Use familiar music to induce recall of autobiographical memories (which may then be shared).** Despite memory impairments, people with dementia are able to retrieve or restore memories, both long term and short term, through familiar music. Often, people with dementia do not recall the details of their autobiographical history (e.g. date of birth, mother's maiden name, year of leaving hometown) *when asked*; however, they are sometimes able to retrieve this information through familiar music and musical activities. In addition, they may experience associations and feelings through the cognitive processing made possible through the music.

## Leading activities for people with dementia: Tips on getting attention—and keeping it

*From staff music therapists, IMNF, "Rhythmic Activities for Everyday Care"*

Remember the following strategies during any kinds of activities or interactions when you want to maintain attention from people with dementia, either as a group or individually!

### Cueing

A cue is the same thing as a reminder. It draws attention to what's happening and to what is to be done. During activities try different forms of cues.

- Visual—any type of cue that the patient can see

  - Make eye contact

- – Make large gestures or movements
- – Point
- – Talk with your hands
- Verbal—any type of cue that is spoken to a patient
  - – Speak loudly
  - – Speak clearly (often this requires you to slow down your normal rate of speaking)
  - – Frequently use the patient's name
  - – Face patient when speaking
  - – Make eye contact when speaking
- Tactile—any type of intervention that involves touch
  - – Lightly touch patient on the arm
  - – Rhythmically tap on the patient's knee
  - – Hold or shake patient's hand
- Cognitive—any type of cue that might spark memory or thought
  - – A familiar song, for example "Happy Birthday"
  - – A familiar rhythm, for example "shave and a haircut"
  - – A familiar sound, for example the doorbell sound or whistling

## Interrupting expectations

When you interrupt the expectations of a patient, often this results in drawing attention to the present moment. Some examples are below.

- Unexpected silence—make a break in sound during an activity
  - – Stop speaking (unexpectedly)
  - – Pause a recording (unexpectedly)
- Unexpected movements—begin or stop movement during an activity
  - – Freeze in an unlikely position (unexpectedly)
  - – Jump, wave, dance
- Unexpected sounds—make a sound during an activity

- Clap (unexpectedly)

- Make a strange mouth noise like "zzzzzzz" or "brrrrrrrrr" (unexpectedly)

- Click your tongue

- Fake an accident (e.g. dropping papers on the floor)

Overall, *present* yourself! You are important, you are a leader. Be one! Remember to command and move the energy, notice the space you are in and maximize it, and have fun!

---

## Music for physical and motor issues

Physical losses and handicaps of all kinds are common among older people. These physical issues tend to have a greater than usual impact on patients with dementia, because of their cognitive impairments. People with dementia lack perceptual motor coordination, or body awareness; in some cases, motor issues result in slurred or unintelligible speech (a condition called dysarthria, which we discuss in Module 8). More commonly, people with dementia experience the physical effects of agitation, tension, and sleeplessness.

Emotional and social problems also affect the ability of people with dementia to address and overcome physical challenges. For example, emotional withdrawal may make it less likely that a person with dementia will feel motivated to make purposeful movements, *or move at all.*

Music is helpful in overcoming inertia, depression, and impediments to movement and speech in people with dementia. Here are some ways to encourage movement:

- Use music to accompany exercise, in therapeutic recreation programs and at home. For people with dementia, as for others, music is a powerful motivator for engaging in group exercise.

- Music therapists know that "feeling the groove" of familiar or improvised music leads to spontaneous movement. That is, listening and feeling the steady beats of music played by a therapist or music partner seems to trigger an internal sense of the beat in people with dementia, as well as others. Use steady beats to engage people with dementia in music. Often, patients who are initially reluctant to participate will hear the beat and become easily motivated and spontaneously engaged in the music.

- **Remember that moving with the music means more than going along with the beat. It means *responding to changes in the music*—** letting the music move you, so to speak.

  - To facilitate this response, music therapists introduce variations in the music, including changes in dynamics, the addition or variation of harmonic texture, or introduction of fragmented notes or rhythmic variation to the initial basic beats. The goal is for patients to feel the music and respond spontaneously, with *expressive* movement.

  - Visual cues, such as the therapist using hands or head movements to signal or exaggerate the rhythmic or dynamic changes, help bring patients into the music.

- People with dementia benefit from making music with simple rhythm instruments such as hand drums, shakers, maracas, tambourines, floor drums, and wrist bells. Playing an instrument involves multi-sensory feedback, and it involves multiple areas of the brain. For example, when a person plays a tambourine, that person hears music, and uses their body to strike forth more music; this energizes the person to keep up with the music, to plan for the beat. Even tapping the tambourine or some other rhythm instrument as it sits in their lap helps a person feel vibrations and come on board with the music. And this is important when there are few felt experiences that engage the person at this level.

  Playing an instrument may also help improve coordination, and hand skills that are useful in daily activities—for example, using flatware or gripping a walker.

Here are some other music interventions that you can deliver, with guidance from a music therapist, to increase muscle strength, endurance, and circulation among your patients with dementia:

- To encourage deep breathing, play arpeggios (the notes of a chord, played one after the other, in ascending or descending order). Breathing in concert with arpeggios helps patients rhythmically inhale, hold their breath, and exhale—leading to therapeutic deep breathing.

- To facilitate stretching, play sounds that mimic and motivate the movement of parts of the body. For example, an ascending rolled chord may facilitate the raising of a shoulder and other therapeutic movements.

- When providing rhythm instruments to a group, create a situation in which group members must move in order to access the instrument or make a sound. This increases a sense of agency, and may help group members communicate rhythmically with one another.

- Institute a circle dance. Begin by moving shoulders to a beat; ask one person to show a dance move; and have the group follow and go around a circle, so that all group members can demonstrate a move, as seen in the accompanying video at www.imnf.org/mhp-book-resources.

- Use rhythm patterns to bring closure to the session. For example, end the session with a drum improvisation, so that group members experience a rhythmic, dynamic, and spontaneous effect of the music as a send-off.

## Therapeutic drumming circles for people with dementia

One of the most effective and popular music interventions for people with dementia is the therapeutic drumming circle, which is described in Module 2. As noted, drumming circles may include all members of the community—people with dementia, depression, and other neurological conditions, as well as caregivers, healthcare staff, and others. That said, many long-term care facilities offer therapeutic drumming circle programs expressly designed to serve people with dementia. These programs are generally open to people with dementia at all levels of functioning—even those who are in late-stage dementia, and those who have little or no motor activity. (Only people who are exhibiting violence or very disruptive behavior are by necessity excluded.) Participating in a therapeutic drumming circle allows people with dementia to respond to one another with feelings of competence "in the moment," and often with joy.

The main challenge in leading a drumming circle for people with dementia is in getting the attention of participants, and maintaining attention over the course of the session. The IMNF has identified best practices for engaging people with dementia in therapeutic drumming and other rhythmic activities.

> To access a sequence from the IMNF therapeutic drumming circle for people with dementia and their caregivers in a skilled nursing facility, visit www.imnf.org/mhp-book-resources.

## Choruses for people with dementia and their caregivers

We began this module by introducing The Unforgettables, a chorus group made up of people with dementia and their family caregivers. This chorus reflects a growing trend to include people with dementia in activities that offer shared experiences in the arts, in a welcoming or "normalized" environment. The early model for this type of program was "Meet Me at MOMA," a special initiative at the Museum of Modern Art, in New York City. The project, which took place from 2007 to 2014, set out to make art and the museum experience accessible to people with Alzheimer's. This was a radically new idea—and it worked. The experience offered real benefits both to people with dementia and their family caregivers.

Mary Mittleman, who founded The Unforgettables, hypothesized that "making music together, rehearsing and giving concerts, might provide even greater benefits than a museum visit, as people with dementia and their family members would work together to create a joyful experience for themselves and their audiences" (Mittleman & Papayannopoulou, 2018, p.779). And this was so.

Bringing people with dementia together in culture-based activities, in an environment that was free of stigma, was a new idea. But singing has long been recognized as therapeutic for people with Alzheimer's as well as other neurological problems.

**Studies of choral programs for seniors in general show that singing together contributes to increased feelings of self-esteem and competence among participants, while providing welcome opportunities for social interaction and stimulation. People with dementia—who ordinarily have few opportunities for social interaction—can join in.** Because people with dementia can often recall familiar lyrics—and even learn new lyrics—singing in a chorus calls on existing abilities, creating a pathway for expression and communication.

Not surprisingly, participation in a chorus tends to improve mood and reduce depression symptoms among people with dementia. In the physical domain, singing under the guidance of a music therapist or choral leader has the potential to improve breathing, posture, and speech as well. Many of these benefits are also experienced by caregivers, who are equal partners in singing, from practice to performance.

In recent years, we've seen a blossoming of community choruses for people with dementia and their family caretakers—not only (or mainly) in the US but also in the UK, Australia, and Canada. Those who are interested in joining or starting a dementia chorus or choir can find robust online information, tools, and resources; to explore the possibilities, visit www.imnf.org/mhp-book-resources.

Although singing groups for people with dementia and their caregivers fall within the interests of music therapists and other clinicians, the choruses have developed outside clinical and senior care settings (though occasionally in partnerships with them). A possibility for the future is to establish comparable choruses within senior care settings, for people with dementia and caregiving staff; such choruses might operate as part of the music therapy program, or as an adjunct to arts-based creative aging activities.

## Familiar songs—yes, it's brain science!

People who care for people with dementia are sometimes amazed to see that patients who no longer recognize their loved ones can still remember the songs, and the words to songs, heard long ago. The familiar song gives these patients pleasure, and sense of who they are. In some cases, patients with dementia are able to learn new songs, and new lyrics, when, it seems, they are unable to learn anything else. As Oliver Sacks (2007, p.337) has said, "Music of the right kind can serve to orient and anchor a patient when almost nothing else does."

### How familiar songs work

We don't entirely know why familiar songs are uniquely effective with people with dementia. But emerging brain science provides hypotheses, or suggestions. It seems that music memories are preserved in the brain, even as other memories are lost. As a result, the response to music may be preserved, even when dementia is very advanced.

Why does this happen? It seems that the brain areas involved in music processing (and music memory) are *preferentially spared* by dementia. These areas are not as affected by the disease as other areas are. Or when they are affected, it doesn't matter quite as much, because there are other brain areas that can partly fill in—areas of the brain that will still respond to music, if music is offered.

When we listen to music, it is processed in many different areas of the brain. There is no one "music center" that might be disabled or compromised. Quite the opposite: there are numerous brain systems that respond to particular musical experiences and skills—and these are distributed throughout the brain.

# How Music Affects Your Brain
## This is how music stimulates different parts of your brain

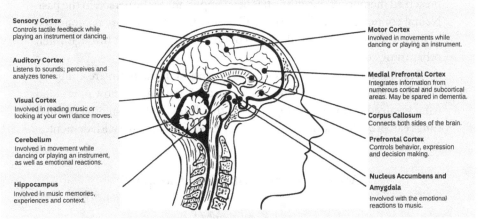

**Sensory Cortex**
Controls tactile feedback while playing an instrument or dancing.

**Auditory Cortex**
Listens to sounds; perceives and analyzes tones.

**Visual Cortex**
Involved in reading music or looking at your own dance moves.

**Cerebellum**
Involved in movement while dancing or playing an instrument, as well as emotional reactions.

**Hippocampus**
Involved in music memories, experiences and context.

**Motor Cortex**
Involved in movements while dancing or playing an instrument.

**Medial Prefrontal Cortex**
Integrates information from numerous cortical and subcortical areas. May be spared in dementia.

**Corpus Callosum**
Connects both sides of the brain.

**Prefrontal Cortex**
Controls behavior, expression and decision making.

**Nucleus Accumbens and Amygdala**
Involved with the emotional reactions to music.

*Figure 4: Music on the mind*

Broadly speaking, dementia tends to result from progressive damage to the areas in the higher brain, or cerebral cortex, and in a lower or subcortical structure called the hippocampus, which is responsible for forming new memories.

The *cerebral cortex* is made up of the right and left brain hemispheres that we are all familiar with. The cortex is responsible for learning and thinking, for language, and for the many kinds of human intelligence and creativity. The cerebral cortex is also responsible for our memories of facts, and information, all the things we consciously "know."

Beneath the cortex are *subcortical brain structures*, which are involved in more basic or "primitive" functions, such as motor control, body temperature, breathing, eating, sleep, sex, and so on. The subcortical structures include the limbic system, which can record memories that are agreeable or disagreeable, and which are felt as emotions, such as pleasure or fear. The hippocampus is part of this system. Functional brain imagery shows that the hippocampus is involved in memory for music and musical experiences.

The higher and lower parts of the brain operate together through numerous neural interconnections. For example, when we listen to music, subcortical structures register our emotional reactions, and the associated memory-feelings that are recorded in this part of the brain. At the same time, neural connections to the cortex (the prefrontal cortex and the auditory cortex) allow us to listen at a different and higher level—to recognize, learn about, and fully experience the music, as part our conscious, thinking life.

*But what if much of the cortex is damaged, as in dementia?*

In that case, the subcortical system provides a backup. The music will register in the subcortical brain, as pleasurable, for example, or as part of a preserved memory, if this music has been important to the person in the past. Neural connections to the cortex will ensure that the memory is supported to the extent possible in the damaged brain. Familiar songs get through when other things don't.

The questions about how music is processed in the brain are complex, exciting, and the subject of ongoing research. But what we know now—and what we need to know as caregivers—is that listening to or singing familiar songs can provide emotional and memory benefits to people with dementia.

## My soundtrack with Glen Campbell

*by Kim Campbell*

A great movie soundtrack sets the tone and personality of a film, making it both recognizable and memorable. Consider how upon hearing only a few notes of any John Williams score; whether it is the awe-inspiring other-worldly *ET*, the courageous and rambunctious *Indiana Jones*, or the futuristic and rebellious *Star Wars*, we instantly remember the film, its characters, and the thrilling journey it took us on.

My late husband, music legend Glen Campbell, and I shared a thrilling journey of our own. The music he made during his more than 50 years as a Grammy winning recording artist ("By The Time I Get To Phoenix," "Galveston," "Southern Nights," and "Wichita Lineman," to name a few) provided a soundtrack not only for "Our Movie" but for millions of people around the world.

As with any great love story, we faced forces that threatened to tear us apart. By the grace of God, we overcame Glen's battle with alcoholism only to face our greatest challenge when Glen was diagnosed with Alzheimer's disease in 2011.

In light of such devastating news, Glen could have retired his guitar and gone into seclusion: but he did just the opposite. He courageously went public with his diagnosis and invited filmmakers James Keach (*Walk the Line*) and Trevor Albert (*Groundhog Day*) to accompany him on a world tour, which was to be the final crescendo of his stellar career.

Accompanied by his band—which included our daughter Ashley on banjo, our son Cal on drums, and our son Shannon on guitar—Glen completed a tour that lasted almost two years, with 151 sold-out shows.

With the aid of a teleprompter for lyrics, he sang from the heart, infusing each song with profound emotion and poetic phrasing. His guitar solos needed no memory aid. They flowed flawlessly from his fingertips as if they were heaven sent. As our son Cal jokingly put it, "Glen could play guitar better than anyone else in the business, with half his brain tied behind his back!"

As the disease began to take its toll, Glen could easily become confused, agitated, or obstinate, sometimes right before a show. But the moment he heard Ashley's banjo play the intro to "Gentle on My Mind," a spark of lucidity returned to his eyes and Glen Campbell was back. When he, the seasoned performer, stepped onto the stage, the world witnessed the miracle of music and memory.

Music brought Glen joy, meaning, and purpose. Timeless songs such as "Amazing Grace" gave him a way to express his faith, and brought him inner peace. He loved to be where the light of music, the light of love, and the light of God was shining on him, like a "Rhinestone Cowboy."

Glen's Goodbye Tour culminated in the 2014 award-winning documentary, *Glen Campbell: I'll Be Me*, a Country Music Association Award, an Oscar nomination, and two Grammys, one of which was for best soundtrack!

Glen's neurologist, Dr. Hart Cohen of Cedars-Sinai Medical Center, said he had no doubt that Glen's persistence in the musical arena helped to preserve his intellectual function far longer than would otherwise have been expected. In the end, music lifted our family's spirits and gave us ways to connect with Glen when words no longer could.

After personally witnessing the remarkable benefits Glen experienced through music, I was inspired to create the Kim & Glen Campbell Foundation as a vehicle to raise funds needed to support research initiatives that seek to understand the therapeutic value of music.

There is an undeniable power to music which spans all cultures, all history, and all time. It is my hope that music's power may be more fully understood and harnessed to benefit those suffering from maladies such as neurological diseases, depression, PTSD, chronic pain, or simply those of us interested in enhancing our own health and well-being.

Downloadable HANDOUT at www.imnf.org/mhp-book-resources.

# Music for Everyday Care of People with Dementia, and Others

*Sing while you comb hair, play music during bath time*
*Hum when putting a patient in bed for the evening.*

Institute for Music and Neurologic Function, 2007

In Module 5, we explored the ways in which music interventions can help people with dementia in assisted living and other residential care settings. As we have seen, one way to deliver music interventions is through group sessions, led by a music therapist, recreation therapist, a specially trained CNA, or a musician volunteer. To participants, this is a "music group." For the group leader, the focus is on achieving therapeutic goals, such as increased self-awareness, social interaction among participants, or improved memory and attention.

Research, and decades of clinical experience, show that therapeutic music groups improve the quality of life for people with dementia, in the emotional, social, and cognitive domains. But here's the rub: group sessions meet once, perhaps twice, and rarely three times a week—for 45 minutes. But most of the challenges in dementia care—the behavioral and psychological symptoms of dementia—show up in daily care situations.

For example, many people with dementia exhibit agitation and anxiety in the late afternoon or early evening; others are resistant and aggressive during morning care. Music interventions have great potential to address these issues. But group music sessions are almost never scheduled in early morning or evening hours. And they don't address intimate care issues. So we need to find a way to bring the power of music to everyday care.

## Caregiver interventions

The person who is most likely to be present when a person with dementia experiences agitation or emotional distress is the frontline caregiver, a family member, CNA, or HHA. Our experience shows that frontline caregivers are well able to use music to reduce the stresses that affect the lives of their patients, *and* the work of caregiving.

In fact, leaders in the field of senior care have come to see the frontline caregiving staff as a valued resource in providing music interventions. David Gentner, President and CEO of Wartburg, which is home to the IMNF, has led the way in including music therapists and other creative arts therapists as part of the dementia healthcare team. At the same time, Gentner recognizes that it is the frontline caregivers who have a first-hand understanding of the challenges that a particular individual—their patient—experiences from day to day. Frontline caregivers are in a position to provide hands-on music interventions that improve the quality of daily care.

A large study of dementia care in the UK reached similar conclusions (Bowell & Bamford, 2018). While recognizing the important role of trained professionals, such as music therapists, the researchers found that some kinds of music interventions were best delivered by frontline caregivers. As examples, it is the CNA or HHA who will know how to engage a patient with a song during their morning routine, or how to use a personalized playlist effectively at bath time. It is the CNA or HHA who is best able to anticipate the onset of agitation or a depressed mood in the patient.

In senior care settings, it is worth noting that CNAs are likely to be the only staff members who engage with patients, *one-on-one*, regularly, *multiple times a day*. As such, they have a unique opportunity to use music in addressing patients' daily needs.

For all of these reasons, CNAs are being trained to use music therapy techniques with their dementia patients. This trend will likely continue. Research shows that CNAs as well as patients benefit from music interventions. Caregivers report that music makes it easier, and more rewarding, to communicate with patients, and move the day's activities along.

One caregiver who uses music therapy says, "It's not just the resident... It lifts my mood as well" (Bowell & Bamford, 2018, p.39).

## Getting started

**No specialized music skills are required to use music in caregiving: anyone who has enjoyed music, as part of their own daily life, can learn to engage their patients through music. Anyone who has been a caregiving parent**

**knows how to "Sing while you comb hair, play music during bath time..."** (IMNF, 2007).

This module will introduce you to evidence-based music therapy techniques that can be delivered by CNAs, HHAs, and other frontline caregivers to improve the quality of life for their patients, and bring new joy and meaning to caregiving.

## ABOUT YOU

### Do you use music as part of your daily routine?
We invite you to take part in this self-questionnaire. Check the boxes that describe the ways you use music in your daily activities. Think about WHY you use music in the ways you do. Fill in the blanks if you feel like doing so. We have created some typical responses, as prompts for your thoughts and responses.

**I use music...**

_____ To wake up (because _____)
*"It gets me up and moving—automatically!"*

_____ While I walk the dog or do my morning power walk (because _____)
*"It paces me, makes me feel healthy and able to meet the day."*

_____ In the car, while I am driving (because _____)
*"Driving is kind of boring, and traffic can be stressful...music makes the commute pleasant."*

_____ At work, when I am able to use headphones (because _____)
*"My music gives me space and privacy in the office situation; I can tune out noise, nonsense, and distractions."*

_____ When I exercise at the gym or elsewhere (because _____)
*"I mean, really, how much fun is it to exercise without music?"*

_____ While I am studying or doing computer work at home (because _____)
*"Music is relaxing, and can also be energizing, like when you have to get something done that doesn't require your full attention."*

_____ After work, when I transition into home life (because _____)
*"Don't we all deserve a break? When I get home I put on a bit of music and dance a bit in the kitchen, making dinner—why not?"*

_____ As I take care of kids or others at bedtime (because _____)
*"Bedtime stories and music make the day end right. The same rhymes, the same songs. It's part of the routine."*

_____ To help me fall asleep (because _____)
*"Music can bring peace and love at the end of the day. You don't hear it end."*

---

## TAKEAWAY

Your patients with dementia bring to their current situation a history of daily activities much like your own. Perhaps they too listened to music in order to tune out noise at the office, or to help them relax at the end of the day. Well, noise is often a problem in a senior residence; and agitation often increases at bed time. Reviewing your own daily use of music may help you meet the needs of your dementia patients, whose needs for music are much like your own.

---

## Background: Caregiving and music over the life span

Caregiving involves attending to, and meeting, the needs of another person for whom we have responsibility. For some of us caregiving becomes a life's work and a profession. But it's a role that all of us can identify with. In the UK, CNAs and home health aides are called "carers." Haven't we all been "carers" at one time or another? Yes, and yes. And haven't we also been a person in care? Yes, again.

Every one of us begins our lives in the care of someone else—a mother, a father, or some other adult on whom we are at first entirely dependent. Over the course of our lives, most of us will experience periods of illness, injury, or disability, when we depend on caregiving from family and friends, or from healthcare professionals and aides.

We know from these experiences that caregiving is *an intimate practice*, touching on the most private moments of our daily life—bathing, dressing, and toileting; eating; walking and moving, with the support of others; sleeping and waking under watchful care. We know, too, that caregiving at its best is personal, involving both "care" and "giving" (and if we are lucky, love as well).

Music, too, is part of the human condition from the very beginning. At all stages of life, music can be an important part of caregiving. Music interventions can help a caregiver meet a person's most basic needs, such as getting dressed in the morning, as well as higher needs, such as needs for belongingness and self-esteem. So we need to bring music into caregiving, to help those who are struggling with dementia *and* the caregivers who are partners in their struggle.

## What you already know about music and caregiving

Caring for a child—a younger sibling, your own child or someone else's—is a near-universal experience.

**If you have ever cared for a child, you probably know something about using music interventions. You may have used music to help an infant stop fussing and fall asleep; to keep a toddler happily occupied; to open up a conversation with your preteen, and in many other ways.**

**Parents and other adults tend to use music naturally with children—** ***because it works.*** Consider the lullaby, a gentle song that literally lulls an infant to sleep, as she is rocked in the arms of her mother. "Hush Little Baby Don't You Cry" is a well-known example. Like most lullabies, it is a simple melody, repetitive (thus lulling). The sound of the mother's voice, the rhythm of her own breathing as she holds the infant, has a deeply calming effect on the infant, and on the mother as well.

The lullaby is easily adapted to the needs of the toddler, who may be soothed by a song or story chanted at bed time. In fact, the lullaby intervention continues to meet our needs throughout life. Have you ever used soft, soothing, and well-loved music to help you fall asleep after a tense day? Have you ever held the hand of a gravely ill loved one, and softly sung or hummed to them, when speech was not possible?

In the Covid-19 crisis, one New York hospital used remote musicians to pipe in Bach, Brahms, and The Beatles to provide comfort to patients surrounded by masked healthcare workers. This sometimes meant, a doctor said, that "a patient's last minutes of consciousness were embraced with beautiful music." Notice the use of the touch-related word "embrace," which calls to mind the mother holding her infant as she sings.

**Consider, as well, the many ways that we naturally use music to "manage" the behavior of young children.** When a child is agitated or bored on a long car trip, we put on a favorite song, one the child will sing along with, and ask us to play again and again. If children are rambunctious on the camp bus, the counselor will get them singing "The Wheels on the Bus" or some other rousing and repetitive song. If the sitter is having trouble administering a night-time medicine, she may wave the spoon about, cheerfully, to the tune of "A Spoonful of Sugar," in which case the sugar may be optional...

You get the point: in each of these examples, music helps the caregiver meet the needs of the child "in a most delightful way." If you have cared for a child, you probably know how to do that.

These music interventions—and many more that we will suggest—can be adapted to help you meet the needs of people with dementia. But before we go forward we need to make one thing clear: in this introduction, we have used examples from childcare *only because* these interventions are most familiar, and natural to us. In no way do we mean to suggest that people with dementia are "like children," because they are not. People with dementia have experienced decades of life in which they have formed a personal history and identity, and have reached levels of cognitive achievement well beyond what children can attain. Not all of that past experience is available to them now. But we can offer a music intervention that meets people with dementia where they are at this moment. Music interventions are adapted to our needs across the life span.

The lullaby lulls the infant to sleep; it may also bring peace and respite to a person at the end of life. The intervention, in both cases, is deeply respectful of the person.

## Using music to meet the challenges of dementia care

CNAs and HHAs are responsible for providing basic care for people living with dementia in a way that respects their individuality and needs. Key challenges for CNAs occur when people with dementia are unable or unwilling to accept care that is offered in support of their health and safety. Music interventions can help the CNA meet the needs of a person with dementia when challenges arise in daily care.

Specifically, music interventions can help to:

- reduce agitation

- support ambulation

- bring ease and pleasure to activities of daily life, including:

  - bathing and personal hygiene

  - dressing

  - toileting

  - eating

  - sleeping and waking behavior

- facilitate participation/cooperation in medical care (including wound care, medication regimes)

- overcome social apathy and withdrawal

- motivate participation in exercise and movement programs

- promote stimulation and enjoyment on resident units.

Music interventions also help CNAs, HHAs, and other caregivers to:

- communicate with people with dementia, so as to better understand their needs

- provide care on a schedule that can be well managed, within a person-centered care environment.

In addition, music interventions contribute directly to the well-being of CNAs and other staff, in ways that have been well documented.


## Music as part of person-centered care

In this module, we will look at the ways that music interventions can support everyday care as provided by CNAs and other caregivers.

We would be happy to know that a caregiver's singing made a person with dementia more cooperative with morning washing and dressing routines. We might be deeply relieved if the music provided in the course of daily care resulted in less aggressive behavior, less screaming, and less distress from those in our care.

But if we are using music in the context of person-centered care, patient cooperation and compliance are not all we aspire to. We will want our patients to be active participants or partners in their care.


### A "music vocabulary"

Music words seem appropriate in describing some of the ways that caregivers and people with dementia can become partners in everyday care.

If caregiving goes well, we might say that:

- the patient is "attuned" to the caregiver (and the music)

- she is "in time" or "in sync" with the CNA and others

- she is "in harmony" with her caregivers much of the time. When there is tension (or dissonance), we are able to use communication—including music and touch—to work toward a harmonic resolution.

As we consider music interventions we will use words like "attuned" and "in time" to describe the outcomes we desire for people with dementia and their caregivers.

## Why music interventions work: It's about rhythm

The music interventions that are most helpful in caring for people with dementia are *rhythmic activities* of one kind or another. Rhythmic activities include rhythmic singing, chanting, clapping, stomping feet, drumming, dancing, and many other movements that are performed to a steady beat that is easy to follow.

Moving rhythmically comes naturally to us, because in a sense "rhythm is us." Our pulse, our heartbeat, our breathing are rhythmic. Our movements are rhythmical, though we are seldom conscious of this: in fact, rhythm makes it possible for us to perform many complex movements *automatically*. Often when we falter, it is because we have lost our inner rhythm, through injury or illness. In music therapy we use rhythm, and rhythmic activities, to restore lost functions, to stimulate and heal.

It's easy to see why rhythmic activities are a powerful therapeutic tool. The first thing we hear, well before we are born, is the steady heartbeat of our mother. And the first movements we make are rhythmical as well. Jacques D'Amboise, the renowned dancer and educator, has said that life begins in a fluid rhythmic dance, within the body of the mother. The mother walks her walk, and the unborn child moves with her rhythm, to the sound of her heartbeat. This rhythmic movement—this dance, if you will—becomes part of life—everyone's life—and we reach back to this experience, as a deep inner resource, as we deal with the challenges and adversities that life hands us.

Research shows that rhythmic activity has a powerful therapeutic effect on people of all ages—from premature infants in the neonatal intensive care unit, to people with dementia in the last stages of the disease. When people with dementia can no longer speak—even when they no longer recognize their own children—they can participate in drum circles, coming together with others to create rhythms as part of a group, and in expression of their own inner rhythms. At all stages of life, and at all stages of dementia, rhythm is us.

## Rhythm is Us

Mickey Hart, the Grateful Dead drummer, has a mission—to show how the rhythmic manipulation of sound can be used for health and healing. All of his work rests on a simple principle:

> Our bodies are multidimensional rhythm machines, with everything pulsing in synchrony, from the digesting activity of our intestines to the firing of neurons in the brain.
>
> Within the body, this main beat is laid down by the cardiovascular system, the heart and the lungs. The heart beats between 60 and 80 times per minute, and the lungs fill and empty at about a quarter of that speed, all of which occurs at an unconscious level.
>
> As we age, however, these rhythms can fall out of sync, and then there is no more important or crucial issue than regaining that lost rhythm. (Hart, 1991, pp.23–25)

### Rhythmic activities in caregiving

Everyone responds to a regular beat, as conveyed by sound or touch: *it is almost impossible not to*. The response occurs in the moment, naturally. Rhythmic activities, then, offer a unique opportunity for caregivers and patients to *respond together* to a stimulus—the musical beat. Being in sync, and attuned to the music, creates a shared experience that is often pleasurable, and also therapeutic.

**The goal for the caregiver is to blend rhythmic activities into everyday acts of care:** "Sing while you comb hair, play music during bathing time... Hum when putting the resident to bed for the evening" (IMNF, 2007).

**As you sing, the steady beat of the song or chant, and the rhythmic movements of your body and hands as you provide care, will help you and your patient move in time, in sync, to complete the activity at hand.**

The music offers something beyond words. "It's like a communication that you never knew you had" (Hsu *et al.*, 2015, as cited in Bowell & Bamford, 2018, p.32).

## "Happy Birthday" gets the job done

During the Covid-19 crisis of 2020, 260 million Americans needed a simple way to protect themselves and their loved ones from infection. They were told to wash their hands—often, and well.

Public health officials found a way to make sure that the job was done thoroughly. They made handwashing a rhythmical activity—a kind of musical intervention. They said, hey, when you wash your hands, sing a song. Sing "Happy Birthday to You," and when you are done with that song, you will know that your hands are clean.

So millions of Americans went to their bathroom sinks and office rest rooms and sang "Happy Birthday" to themselves as they washed their hands. These singers in the washroom were adults as well as children. They were not under an illusion that they were celebrating anyone's birthday; but the song, the music, the rhythm helped them pace themselves, to comply with an important health regimen. That's one way that music interventions work. For everybody.

## Selecting music for caregiving

A first step in using music in caregiving is to become familiar and comfortable with the music that is most likely to engage the person with dementia.

- Review the personal playlist of the person with dementia, if they have one (see "Using pre-recorded music: Personalized playlists" in Module 5). The playlist will include music that is well loved and personally meaningful to your patient. Not all of these selections will be appropriate for use in a given care activity: for example, a song that was shared with a beloved partner, recently deceased, might not be a good choice for bath time or exercise. On the other hand, a theme from a favorite action movie or TV show might work very well. A music therapist or recreation therapist can help you identify songs on the patient's playlist that may lend themselves to daily care activities.

- The patient's personalized playlist will also tell you *what kind of music* the patient responds to: country, jazz, rock and roll, classical, and so on. The selections may suggest songs from your own repertoire of favorites, which you might sing or play on an iPod during care activities.

- When using songs in daily care, there is no reason to feel restricted to songs on the patient's playlist (as you might if you were addressing memory or emotional issues). Choose music that is simple, rhythmical, and similar to the music that your patient enjoys. And just as important, *choose music that you enjoy*. Think about developing your own personal playlist, as a resource for yourself, going forward.

- Include music that reflects the many rhythms of caregiving. As you review your patient's playlist, or develop a playlist of your own, try to identify:

  - chant-like music that is mainly rhythmical, without much emotional content. This will help move the patient in sync with a care activity. Check the playlist: It is most effective to use songs that the patient knows

  - "wake up" music. This may arouse the patient and elicit participation in a care activity, such as dressing or bathing

  - "dance-like" music with a strong and swinging beat, such as a song in waltz meter (e.g. 1, 2, 3/1, 2, 3) or early rock and roll. Dance-like rhythms may stimulate movement across a variety of daily activities, including ambulation and exercise

  - "wind-down" music—soft, slow, or lulling music; this may relax the patient, bring the patient in sync with a care activity, and reduce anxiety. Slow music also works well as a background during dining and at bedtime.

## Guidance for family care partners

Family members play an important role in putting together a personal playlist for a loved one with dementia. When family members are care partners, they can be very effective in using music selections in therapeutic ways: to lift the mood of the person with dementia, elicit pleasurable memories, encourage participation in family life, and more. *But there's a challenge*—because family care partners typically have lived many years with their loved one, and know them well, they tend to become upset when a musical selection fails to have the expected response. They may feel defeated, *even rejected*, when a favorite song fails to bring comfort and emotional closeness. They wonder what they have done wrong.

It is worth putting this last response in a larger context: communication often goes off course between loved ones, even in the absence of neurological problems. For example, a joke that a family member often makes about their loved one's endearing mishaps usually binds them together, in mutual acceptance and understanding. But maybe not if the loved one has had a very bad day at the office. In that case, the familiar rhythm and music of the back-and-forth is disrupted. The loved one is irritated, and ready to retreat. The family care partner learns to quickly turn to a comfort mode.

It's not so different when using music to communicate with a loved one who has dementia. Much-loved music may become irritating or ineffective if the person has an undiagnosed pain (even a dull pain), is sleep deprived, or is experiencing fear or anxiety in response to a medical or social interaction. When the familiar rhythm and music of the back-and-forth is disrupted, it's not a crisis. It just means that one partner (the care partner) must turn quickly to the comfort mode. That might mean a gentle touch, in the way long favored, a reduction in stimulation from music and other sources (e.g. noise, and company), and communication in the way that has come to serve the care partner and their loved one, at this time in their lives together.

In the case of the person with dementia, a negative response to a favorite song may indicate a state of physical discomfort or pain that the person is unable to communicate in words. It is important to try to discover the source of the physical distress, if any, as a first step.

- If words do not help, it can be worth trying a gentle touch where the care partner thinks their loved one might be experiencing pain. The care partner could touch their head, knee, shoulder, belly, or other part of their body that might be hurting.

- There may be other reasons for pain. Does the loved one have a new health problem, such as constipation or toothache? Has a chronic condition such as arthritis flared up? The care partner should consult the healthcare team if their loved one continues to reject usual sources of comfort and pleasure, including music from the personalized playlist that is part of their caregiving.

If the person does not seem to be in pain or physical distress, it is worth considering the possibility that the musical selection played is too stimulating, or in other respects insensitive to the person's mood at the moment. For example, if the loved one with dementia is at this moment fearful and withdrawn, a musical favorite that begins with a rousing introduction may cause further withdrawal. If the loved one seems at this moment to be emotionally present in unexpected ways—sadder or more hostile to the care partner or the situation—a romantic song that is usually shared happily may lead to "anger" or distress. Communication can be restored if the care partner can turn to a comfort mode, such as they have established over the years, and for now.

The personal playlist is a powerful tool that can help family care partners care for, and communicate with, their loved ones. What the playlist cannot easily do is restore the familiar music and rhythm of communication between loved ones. That's because it is the care partner who responds by providing comfort when communication goes off course; but the person with dementia cannot respond in the same way, as they used to do—and that is a great loss to the care partner.

Music therapists can help care partners in their efforts to communicate with their loved ones with dementia, and, so far as possible, restore the rhythmic and musical back-and-forth that is part of communication in a close relationship.

For the person with dementia who does not have a personalized playlist, the care partner can use the form (see "Music assessment questionnaire" in Module 5) to identify their music preferences. They can also use this form to review their own favorite music, which will be an important resource to them in caregiving.

## Caregiver singing

Singing is a way of communicating with the person you care for: your child, your ailing spouse, your aging parent, your patient.

**Here's what you need to know about singing with your patients with dementia:**

- **When you sing, use not just your voice, but your whole body**, to communicate nonverbally, through music and rhythm.

    - Move your head and upper body expressively, as you sing. And if you are moving across the room, for example, walk in time to the music. This will happen naturally if you are attuned to the music. Dance steps may also be a possibility for some caregivers.

    - **Eye contact with your patient is critically important.** Do not sing if you are engaged in a task that requires you to look continuously at equipment, a paper form, or a sheet of lyrics.

    - If you are handling clothes or other items as part of care, try holding them before you at near-eye level, as you would a microphone, and keep eye contact with the patient. Sing to your patient.

- It helps if you think of singing as a form of *nonverbal* communication, quite different from ordinary speech. Yes, when you sing, you are saying words: but you are not talking, you are singing. **The words in your song—the verbal content—may or may not be meaningful to**

**your dementia patients.** The words are embedded in music, and it is the music that gets through, to deliver a therapeutic experience. Songs can be hummed. They can be composed without words, for instruments or ensembles—in which case a composer may call them "airs," "arias," or even "songs without words." You can use songs to communicate, with or without words, in your caregiving.

- **Feel free to hum songs, in whole and part, as you help your patients in their daily activities.** Humming can help you keep the music going when you don't have time to find words or prepare a complete song. For most of us, humming comes naturally from our own inner music and rhythm. It's often a form of self-soothing, for example in busy or harassing situations, and tends to be comforting to patients.

- **You can substitute song-like syllables, such as "la, la, la" for words**, especially in expressive melodies from your patient's culture, where the music meaning is clear. For example, in Jewish music there is a whole genre of melodies (called niguns) sung to "Bim Bam," and "Lai, Lai, Lai." The music provides the emotional message—ranging from joy to lamentation. Melodies, alone, can do that.

- **You can make up songs with minimal word content.** For example, try engaging your patient with dementia by singing "hello, hello," to a lively melody during morning care, and encouraging a song-like response from your patient.

- If you know your patient well, improvise around their name. For example, on entering the room for morning caregiving, you might sing "Hello Carlos," with a rising voice and with gestures, and call for a "Hello" in response. Repeat this over and over again, back and forth, in a song-like way as you initiate caregiving. You can also do playful variations on a patient's name. Eventually, your patient may respond in turn.

- **Touch can also be an important part of the nonverbal communication that is achieved through singing.** Touching your patient's arm as you sing—or marking the beat as you comb hair or wash hands—will help your patient become *attuned* to the care that you are providing, *in time* with the music.

## "You deserve a break today"

Suppose you are a caregiver, assigned to morning care. If you are looking for an ice-breaker—and especially if you don't yet know the personal preferences of your patient—the world of advertising offers many possibilities.

We all know the musical slogans and jingles of mainstream products—we can't avoid them. They are designed to be catchy, and to provide feel-good moments, without meaning anything very specific. They are part of our culture; some of the best-known commercial jingles have been created or sung by popular artists such as Barry Manilow, Justin Timberlake, Bob Marley, and The New Seekers.

This is good news for caregivers. With a few good commercial jingles in your repertoire, you can be pretty sure of making contact with your patients who watch a lot of TV, and may have intact memories of the commercial jingles of the past.

Here are some entry lines, for singing:

- You deserve a break today (McDonald's)

- I'd like to teach the world to sing in perfect harmony (Coca Cola)

- The best part of waking up is Folgers in your cup! (So, hey, let's get going!)

- One love, one heart. Let's get together and feel alright! (Jamaica Airlines)

- I'm Lovin' it! (McDonald's)

- Like a Good Neighbor, [your name] is (t)here (State Farm)

- Double your pleasure, double your fun with Doublemint, Doublemint gum [or anything else you want to insert here!]

- I'm Chiquita Banana and I'm here to say [whatever you want to say!]

- Plop, Fizz. Oh what a relief it is! (Alka Seltzer)

There are many other jingles from past decades that may trigger memories and evoke good feelings.

And, of course, there are new jingles that find their way onto the TVs in day rooms of senior care facilities.

Singing jingles will likely get the attention of your patients, because that's what commercial jingles are designed to do. They are also designed to create good feelings and satisfaction in the product—which in this case is the caregiving at hand.

Try it. You deserve a break today!

### Singing as communication—why it works

We've made the point that caregiver singing is a form of nonverbal communication quite different from ordinary speech. And now we need to say why that is important.

As we have seen, areas of the brain that process music may be preferentially spared in dementia. That means that people with dementia can often sing, or respond to music, when they can no longer understand the words of family members and caregivers.

In people with dementia, the language centers of the brain may be severely compromised. But when words are embedded in music, the brain recruits those areas of the brain that are likely spared, for the processing of music—and your song. The words you sing to your patients may get through to them, when the words you speak are met with confusion or resistance.

Some caregiving activities require a lot of verbal and nonverbal communication between caregivers and patients, if they are to proceed in sync and in harmony. For example, getting washed and dressed requires ongoing prompts or instructions from the CNA: for example, "Let's get ready, and washed; let's put on this shirt, and can you put your arms through, here?" A few studies (e.g. Hammar *et al.*, 2010), and many years of clinical experience, show that caregiver singing (and other music interventions) help people with dementia to better understand these prompts and instructions, and participate in activities of daily care.

Here are some tips and applications—based on a growing body of research:

- **Caregivers can sing or rhythmically communicate with patients about what they are doing, or are about to do.** The verbal communications, which are embedded in music, have a greater chance of being processed and understood than would words alone (for reasons explained above).

  - **Sing your instructions, improvising along the way.** Here's an example, from a caregiver trained in music interventions: "I would be singing, saying, 'We're going to get you washed, here we go today.' And then I'd start into a song, singing their name like... (sings), 'Come on then G [resident], we're going to go G, let's get ready and we'll get washed' (laughs). And then G would look and she'd give a little smile. So it's like a communication that you never knew you had" (Hsu *et al.*, 2015, as cited in Bowell & Bamford, 2018, p.32).

  - When you are singing instructions, for dressing or combing hair for example, **act out these instructions with movements.** (When your patient with dementia sees you demonstrating the activity in this way, they may feel empowered to join in and comb their hair themselves.)

- Use short rhythmic chants and song passages to initiate daily activities. For example, when you walk into a room of a patient who is sleepy or withdrawn, try a simple chant like: "1 o'clock, 2 o'clock, 3 o'clock, 4. If you say you're happy, I'll give you some more." Or sing a "wake up" song, perhaps clapping hands and inviting the patient to join in. Or tap a wake-up rhythm, such as "shave and a haircut," and see if the patient responds.

- Talk in rhythm (rap or sing to a patient) as you wheel them down the hallway (e.g. "We're going, we're going, we're going down to therapy"). Or sing a snippet of a song that the patient is likely to know, such as "We're off to see the Wizard," or "Over the river and through the woods," perhaps improvising words to fit the moment. You might also find a familiar song, with a move-along rhythm, on the patient's personal playlist.

• Caregivers can use familiar and favorite songs (from patients' personal playlists), or traditional songs in their culture, to enhance communication and participation in daily activities. In this approach, the song you choose will *not* relate to the activity at hand, but will evoke other experiences, such as dancing, falling in love, celebrating a holiday, or traveling to faraway places. Many traditional songs and golden oldies can provide pleasurable moments as part of daily care. Songs should be rhythmical and well paced for the activity at hand.

## What to expect when singing is part of everyday care

• More eye contact between you and your patient with dementia; **a sense that your patient is more "present" than usual, more attuned to your presence, and more engaged in the care activity.** As one caregiver put it, "Before it was only me focusing on the situation, now it is both... It is mutual in some way" (Hammar *et al.*, 2010, p.38).

• **Enhanced communication between you and your patient during daily activities.** Your patient's communication may be verbal or non-verbal, and may include:

- singing or humming along with you

- tapping, clapping, or moving in time to the music

- filling in (or making up) the words to a song

- requesting additional songs

- making suggestions or corrections to your singing.

- **Less agitation and confusion in your patient, as a result of enhanced communication.** Screaming and other aggressive behaviors from people with dementia are often rooted in a terrible loss that these patients are experiencing—the loss of the ability to express their needs and fears to those who are close to them. That loss may lead to a kind of panic when they are made to accept intimate care from relative strangers. **Caregiver singing and shared rhythmic activities have been shown to reduce agitation and aggressive behaviors in people with dementia.**

- An easier completion of daily activities, as music provides a way of keeping caregiver and patient in time with one another and the task at hand. Often, in care situations, the CNA initiates a task, with words and instructions, and the person with dementia either does not understand, or cannot move forward in time with the caregiver. The patient seems frozen, as the CNA presses forward, with morning hygiene and dressing—which of course must be completed on schedule. **Caregiver singing and rhythmic chanting help the CNA and the person with dementia to move at the same pace, attuned to each other.** Of course, this results in less resistance, and fewer difficulties.

## Music to prevent agitation and distress

For most frontline caregivers, the greatest challenges come when a patient is in terrible distress. In dementia, distress shows up in many forms, including depression, apathy, and agitation. Among these, agitation presents the most urgent challenge, in part because it sometimes involves aggression and self-harm, and sometimes even harm to caregivers.

For people with dementia, agitation may be expressed in:

- excessive motor activity, such as pacing and rocking; restlessness; and repetitious movements, such as touching a part of the body repeatedly

- abnormal vocalizations, such as wailing or repeating words over and over

- verbal aggression, such as yelling and screaming, and use of profanity

- physical aggression, such as shoving, pushing, and hitting others, and other dangerous and destructive behaviors. (International Association for Music and Medicine, 2020)

Except for pacing, rocking, and repetitive movements, these behaviors are not rhythmic in nature; they are what happens when a person's inner rhythm is out of sync with what is happening to them and around them. They tell us that the person is out of control, due to fear, confusion, frustration, and often anger. The person who is yelling, pushing, or hitting is similarly out of rhythm and out of control.

Music therapists have tended to take a preventive approach to agitation in people with dementia: that is, they use music and rhythmic activities to help people with dementia keep in sync with the caregiving environment, as much as possible, so that agitation and aggression does not reach crisis levels. Music therapists may also help people express their agitation or hyperactivity in the context of music, allowing them to express feelings in a safe environment.

**A growing body of research shows that group music interventions in general are effective in reducing agitated behavior in people with dementia, not just in the group session but over the course of daily care.** For example, one study suggests that a group music intervention program may have reduced "problem behavior," including agitation, by creating a calmer environment and feelings of happiness and relaxation (Lin *et al.*, 2011). There is much anecdotal evidence to support this view.

Although we can't specify the neuropsychiatric roots of agitation in people with dementia, it seems clear that agitation often arises from a patient's inability to communicate verbally, and from confusion and fear as to what is happening as the caregiver approaches. This in turn leads to resistance to care, and sometimes aggression.

As we have seen, singing and other rhythmic activities help caregivers and people with dementia communicate in the course of everyday care, and become more in tune and in time with each other. The practices we have described above are effective in preventing agitation. Using pre-recorded music in the form of personal playlists is another very good option.

## Using personalized playlists to prevent agitation

Personalized playlists for people with dementia have received much attention in recent years, due in part to videos and stories in the media, including public endorsements of this intervention from mainstream organizations such as the Alzheimer's Association, the AARP, and others. Today, many senior care and healthcare organizations offer personalized playlist programs for people with dementia; programs are also available for family caregivers to use at home. An advantage of playlist interventions is that they are pre-recorded, and ready to go, as needed. And it turns out that personal playlist interventions are especially effective in reducing agitation.

A review of the use of music playlists in more than 13 countries, with results from 28 studies, found that "one of the most consistent findings was in relation to agitation," with several studies demonstrating improvements in agitation levels in subjects receiving playlist interventions, as compared to subjects in control groups, who did not (Garrido *et al.*, 2017, p.1139). Researchers noted that some promising results were reported from studies in which frontline caregivers were trained to use the playlists as part of everyday care.

Here are some tips for using personalized playlists to prevent agitation in the course of everyday care:

- With the help of a music therapist, identify music on your patients' personal playlists that has the potential to be engaging and soothing. In general, the music you choose should be of a slow to moderate tempo, with a steady beat, in an arrangement that is familiar to your patient.

- Music that is happy or upbeat can work well, but there is no reason to avoid music that has a sad or contemplative cast. Ballads and folk songs with melancholy words and harmonies may be soothing, because they so often tap into nostalgia and sentiments deeply rooted in identity.

- Reduce erratic environmental noise, distractions, and interruptions before you begin the listening session. Make sure your patient's phone is silenced. If you are participating in the listening experience, make sure your phone is silenced too. Don't let anything destroy the rhythm you want to establish.

- **Be aware of your patient's level of comfort with headphones.** Some people with dementia become anxious or confused when made to wear headphones. An option is to play the music on speakers in the patient's room or other private space.

- **Introduce the music selection before the time of day when your patient typically begins to experience restlessness or other signs of agitation.** Many people with dementia experience restlessness and agitation in the late afternoon or early evening hours; if your patient tends to become agitated around 4:30pm, for example, a playlist intervention at 3:30pm might be most effective.

- If possible, be present during at least part of the listening experience. And check on your patient at regular intervals, beginning within the first 30 minutes of the playlist intervention. Observe how your patient responds to the music. Positive responses from your patients might include them closing their eyes, moving their hands or feet, nodding in time with the music, or humming along. Be especially attuned to any seemingly negative responses, such as a tearful expression or handwringing, or evidence of growing agitation. Although negative responses are relatively uncommon, they may occur, in some cases requiring consultation with the music therapist or the healthcare team. A change of music selection or discontinuation of the playlist intervention may be indicated.

- If the playlist intervention seems to be effective in preventing agitation, try to arrange for your patient to listen to the music selection at about the same time every day, as consistently as possible. (This may require some coordination with other frontline caregiving staff.) The goal is to trigger a response that defuses agitation before it starts.

Why do these music interventions work? Agitation is often experienced when things seem unpredictable and out of control—when the steady beat and rhythm of life is for the moment lost. A music selection that is *predictable and soothing* helps the patient feel safe in the moment; with continued and regular use, the music may become a reliable way of reducing agitation.

## ABOUT YOU

### Reducing agitation on your own

Agitation is very common among people with dementia, affecting up to 70 percent of dementia patients. We might well ask, what percentage of caregivers share in this distress? The answer is 70 percent—or more. Not surprisingly, exposure to dementia-related agitation and aggression is a major cause of caregiver burnout.

It doesn't have to be that way.

Using music, in the ways described above, can help you meet the needs of your patients, and prevent or reduce agitation. At the same time, these music interventions will help meet your needs as a caregiver. It turns out that your needs in this situation are not so different from those of your dementia patient.

So how are you doing?

1. When you have a difficult day, with patients who become resistant or agitated, what do you do to relieve stress?

2. Is music a part of your way of relieving stress? (*Do you put on jazz or country music favorites as you are driving home or making dinner, to wind down? Do you tune into your favorite music as you turn off the lights?*) What's your routine?

_____

3. Do you sometimes make music, as a way of relieving stress (and for pleasure)? (*Do you sing in religious services? Take a turn at karaoke? Pick up a guitar?*) What works for you?

_____

4. Have you developed your own personalized playlist? If so, which musical selections are most effective in relieving stress?

_____

5. Some people are able to imagine music—to play music in their minds—to relieve stress, anxiety, or pain, or to help them move forward in the moment. Have you had an experience in which you were able to play or hear music in your mind, in a way that was helpful to you? If so, can you reference this experience?

_____

_____

## Music to manage pain and physical distress

Pain or discomfort is not an uncommon experience among older people. People with dementia are as likely as others to experience distress from arthritis and joint pain, urinary infections, diabetic neuropathy, and other chronic diseases. But especially in the later stages of dementia, a person might not be able to tell a caregiver or family member about the distress they are experiencing. Yet, if they are to get help, they have to let someone know, somehow.

In this situation, the person with dementia falls back on the behaviors of the preverbal years. Like an infant or preverbal child, they may "make a face," cry, scream, or yell; go rigid, flail about, and even hit those closest to them. We lovingly respect the youngest members of our human family by assuming, *without question*, that the crying, flailing, or hitting is a signal of pain and distress that we must move quickly to relieve. Experts in the care of people with dementia say we must do the same for our dementia patients: "Look for the cause of distress. If not obvious, assume it is due to pain" (CaringKind, 2022, p.15).

Once recognized, pain may be treated with medical and pharmacological interventions. In addition, and over the course of treatment, caregivers are called on to help manage a patient's pain and physical discomfort. Music interventions can be helpful in reducing the experience of pain.

## Using personalized playlists to help manage pain and physical distress

When an infant or preverbal child is experiencing discomfort, caregivers rush to meet the immediate physical need (the bottle or diaper change). In addition, it is natural to provide tactile comfort (holding) and rhythmic comfort (a familiar song or lullaby, a rocking or rhythmic bounce on the lap). People with dementia need the same kind of attention in order to return to a state of relative comfort.

Here are some tips for using personalized playlists to address pain and discomfort in the course of everyday care:

- Become familiar with the ways in which your patient communicates pain and distress. The signals people give vary; as parents will tell you, one baby screams their head off, and another goes rigid and silent. Similarly, people with dementia vary in the way they communicate discomfort to others. If possible, ask family members to tell you how your patient acts when in pain and distress. (They will know.)

- Try a gentle touch if you have reason to believe that that will be helpful. For example, take the patient's hands in yours and sway them, rocking them gently as you hum a familiar song or chant words of comfort.

- Identify selections on your patient's personalized playlist that are pleasurable, and promote relaxation. Introduce these selections when the person is receptive to the intervention; for example, when they have received pain medications or other medical interventions deemed necessary; when there is time and quiet space for comfortable listening.

  - Note that people who are in severe discomfort may be unable to listen to music, even when their preferred music is played. If the music cannot engage their attention, it may be annoying (and the desired effect, of comfort, is not realized). In this situation a caregiver may be able to engage the patient by guiding the listening process (Clair, 1996, p.131). For example, the caregiver or family care partner might say, "I'm here with you. I've brought you your favorite song and I want to listen to it with you." Family care partners will find ways to personalize the suggested script.

- If a person does not respond to recorded music, live singing may be effective in managing pain or discomfort. Caregivers can begin by saying, "I'm going to sing to you now," and proceed to sing the parts of favorite songs that the patient is most likely to be familiar with—the choruses especially. Singing can take place at the bedside in the care setting. Family care partners can identify other appropriate settings. The person with dementia will be invited to sing along, to move with the music (e.g. tap a finger, nod the head—which often happens whether or not it is solicited). This engagement helps the person focus on the music, in the moment, rather than on their pain (Clair, 1996).

• Observe and record the effects of songs and musical selections on the behavior of the person with dementia. Are there selections that seem to reduce pain-related behaviors? If so, make a note of this on the medical record. In some healthcare facilities, nurses, CNAs, and other members of the healthcare team can access information about the use of music as a non-pharmacological means for managing a patient's pain.

(As an example: one facility kept MP3 players with each resident's favorite music on the nursing med cart. For those with chronic pain, the nurse would "administer" the MP3 player, before giving Tylenol. The only challenge was in ensuring that the MP3 players were fully charged—which can easily be done by having devices plugged into a multiple USB charging hub when not in use.)

## Applications to dining and sleeping

Some evidence suggests that playing "relaxing" music during meal times can reduce agitation and aggression among patients with dementia (Chang *et al.*, 2010, as cited in Gentner, 2017; Johnson & Taylor, as cited in Bowell & Bamford, 2018).

Music interventions can also help people with dementia prepare for bedtime and healthful sleep. Sleep is a quality-of-life issue for older people, and not only for them. At every stage of life, sleep affects memory, cognitive capacity, and overall wellness. In older people, lack of sleep increases the likelihood of falls; often contributes to depression; and increases the risks associated with chronic diseases.

**Music has been shown to be effective in inducing sleep in older people. As one study notes, "Slow repetitive rhythms so often can imbue feelings of safety and familiarity that can prepare and induce the brain's sleep response"** (Loewy, 2020, p.2). Familiar music, selected by the person with dementia, provides the most comfort. When music is matched or entrained to breathing rhythms—and these rhythms are repeated over and over again—music may slow the heart rate and reduce night-time anxiety. Music at bedtime also blocks off noise that might otherwise keep a person awake. It appears that people who use music in their everyday activities may derive the most benefit from music that is selected to improve sleep quality.

## Music, moderate or slow? Take a pulse

For people with dementia who experience agitation or anxiety, music therapists often recommend using music with a slow or moderate tempo. The goal is to engage the person with dementia in the music, in a pleasurable, relaxing way. So slow and soothing music is often the best choice.

But what is slow for you or for your patient is of course subjective. So we need guidance on *tempo*, which refers to the overall speed or pace of the music.

Tempo is typically measured by the number of beats per minute (BPM), so you can determine whether a piece of music, as usually played, is "slow" or "moderate."

A general guideline is that a music tempo can be regarded as slow if it is less than about 80 BPM, fast if it is greater than about 120 BPM, and moderate if it falls in between. For reference, the normal pulse rate for an adult is between 60 and 100 BPM. So the music we love is pretty much in time with our normal heartbeat. (No surprise!)

To determine the tempo of music that you may want to use, count the beats in the music per minute, as you would do if you are taking a pulse from a patient. Or clap along with the beats for one minute and note the number of claps you do in that time.

For reference, familiar favorites that are typically performed in a slow tempo (less than 80 BPM) are "Lean on Me" (Bill Withers), 75 BPM, and "My Way" (Frank Sinatra), 75 BPM.

Familiar favorites that are typically performed at a moderate tempo (less than 120 BPM) include "Can't Help Falling in Love" (Elvis Presley), 100 BPM, and "Unforgettable" (Nat King Cole), 113 BPM.

# Music Therapy and Movement Rehabilitation

More than 20 years ago, a few music therapists who worked in nursing homes began to notice that music could have "an almost magical power" on patients with dementia. Patients who were agitated and confused, and unable to communicate, would often respond to familiar music with a slow outpouring of memories and associations...so that it was possible to see the person who was "alive inside." Many of the music therapy best practices that are offered in this guidebook build on our understanding of the transformative effects of music on people with dementia.

Just as magical—but generally receiving less attention—is the power of music to override movement impairments, on the path to rehabilitation. It turns out that music—and more particularly rhythm—helps us draw on areas of the brain that are relatively spared in neurological diseases such as stroke, Parkinson's disease, and brain and spinal cord injuries, so that we move readily to music, even when will and conscious effort fail us.

## The story of Sam

The story of Sam illustrates the power of music to help restore movement after a debilitating stroke (Tomaino, 2002, p.22). Sam was a nursing home resident in his late sixties who was recovering from a stroke. His physical therapist described him as a "guarded walker"—able to shuffle along with a four-footed cane, but not steady enough to walk outside where he might have difficulty negotiating an uneven pavement. Because his left side was weak, his left foot dragged along the floor, causing him to falter. Every step was slow and hesitant, as Sam focused intensely on the process of walking. After he had been in traditional physical therapy for two months, and was showing little further improvement, he was referred to music therapy in the hope that he could improve his sense of his body's position and his balance.

The physical therapist tested Sam's gait, and I, as music therapist, found music with a tempo that matched the pace of his stride. Sam knew the music, and was comfortable walking to it. It reminded him of how, as a teenager, he used to go dancing every week at the gym. As he walked he became more confident of his movements. Amazingly, he began to add dance steps, sliding his feet or clicking his heels! He said he couldn't help it: it just happened.

He wasn't "thinking about walking," he said, he was "thinking about dancing."

After several weeks of twice-weekly sessions, Sam began lifting his left leg off the floor. Now his steps were in perfect time to the rhythm of the music. He was not consciously aware of this, but said that he could feel the tempo in his leg and thought he was able to feel the floor with his left foot. This suggested that he was regaining sensation and control on that side of his body. But when the music stopped, Sam would again shuffle, and drag the affected leg.

What next? As music therapist, I had selected music that Sam knew, so that he would be able to sing to himself, and thus self-cue when he was on his own. Working with the physical therapist, I suggested this as a way to reinforce Sam's therapy in the gym. Recent research has shown that this "internal singing" stimulates the motor areas in the brain. And so, in a range of circumstances—in the gym and on his own—rhythm continued to work as a cue that organized Sam's walking, without his conscious effort.

## TAKEAWAYS

In this module we will see many cases in which an external cue, such as rhythmic music, has a therapeutic effect on motor function. A dance rhythm helps a stroke victim organize his walking; a rhythmic pulse helps a person with Parkinson's disease initiate and improve her gait. All of us respond to such external cues, but this is not a simple or mechanical process. The external cue must be *internalized*; it must be a cue that speaks to something within us, to a past experience of music, dance, or movement, of which we may not be fully conscious. In effect, a rhythm in the external world is heard and *internalized*, evoking an answering rhythm within us. (As Sam said, *he could feel the tempo in his leg.*)

Why was Sam not able to simply will his leg to move as he wished? Most likely the areas of the brain that respond to thoughts of initiating or shaping movement were damaged as a result of the stroke. It turns out that the thought or wish to move depends on higher cortical processing; but the actual ability to move depends on lower (subcortical) brain regions, which are often spared in stroke or neurological disease. The subcortical regions provide a kind of backup for patients like Sam. The musical rhythm reaches these subcortical areas, and activates them, providing a jump start for the motor nerves that are still functional. That's why Sam was able to walk confidently in response to the external rhythmic cue, before the higher cortical areas had been recruited to action.

## Music therapy for movement disorders: The basics

In a subacute rehabilitation unit, the care team works with patients who have lost function after an injury, or in the course of neurologic disease. The cause may be stroke, Parkinson's disease, multiple sclerosis, brain or spinal cord injury, or other traumatic injuries.

The goal is to restore a person to the highest level of function possible, so that they can live as fully and independently as possible, at home. Often what has been lost is the ability to coordinate movement—to move, walk, and speak in a natural way. Often, too, patients have cognitive issues. For example, they may not understand the therapist's instructions or may have problems thinking through the action that they need to do in therapy. Typically, for someone who has had a stroke, thinking of "how to do" something is as much of a problem as the movement itself. Because music provides cues that don't require patients to think about their actions—they just follow the music—music therapy can help those patients who are at risk for extended rehabilitation.

**Music has been shown to be a powerful tool for restoring the mobility of people who have movement disorders.** Strong rhythmic music, prescribed as part of rehabilitation care, can allow people with Parkinson's disease or stroke to regain function—to walk or even dance again. Music-making with adapted instruments can help injured and neurologically disabled people to express themselves in music, while meeting their rehabilitation goals—to increase range of motion, strength, coordination, and balance.

### Rhythm and movement

Oliver Sacks, MD, co-founder of the Institute for Music and Neurologic Function, wrote that "There is in health an implicit music...that is rooted first and foremost in the rhythmicity of all nervous action and its tying together" (1991). We experience this rhythmicity in health, and must work to restore it when we are injured or neurologically impaired.

It's easy to say why this is so. You can't walk, swim, ride a bike, or drive a car unless you do so rhythmically. Have you ever had a significant ankle or leg injury? If so, you will have discovered that you can move forward if, *and only if*, you can establish a new rhythm that allows you to limp or tow your leg along *in an organized way*. If you use crutches, you will need to establish a whole new rhythm, beginning in your arms, and swinging yourself forward. You may find yourself counting rhythmically to get this done—and feeling the new beat of your orthopedic boot or crutches on the ground ahead.

Similarly, when a person suffers neurological damage or disease, their usual rhythms are disrupted in some way. Their inner music is no longer propelling them forward. **Music therapy seeks to restore this inner music, by providing a strong rhythmic pulse from an external source**; this may be provided by a music therapist, either using a drum to establish the rhythmic cue, or using pre-recorded rhythms. Once the correct rhythm is selected, it can be recorded for the patient to use in rehab in between sessions. The music selected will help the patient re-organize their movement going forward, and as they recover.

### Music and movement—an inescapable connection

Music *moves* us, literally. When we listen to music we are moved to feel joy or sadness, excitement or repose, suspense or well-being...through the power of music.

But that's not all. Note that the word "emotion" has within it the word "motion" (it's built on the Latin root, "to move"). It turns out that engaging with music *moves us—literally*. Sometimes we are aware of this: for example, feeling the groove of a familiar tune leads to spontaneous movement, such as foot-tapping. (We can't help it!) More often, we are unaware of the ways that music moves us, because our responses are not observable by ourselves or others. But our physiological responses to music can be observed and measured by biomedical and neuroscience researchers. And what we have learned is that **the ways in which we move to music reflect the "rhythmicity of all nervous action"—the foot-tapping responses of our inner selves. Scientists and music therapists refer to this phenomenon as** *entrainment*, **which means that an external signal, in this case rhythm, is influencing a matching response within our brain.**

- When you listen to live or recorded music, brain imaging will show activity in those areas of your brain that are related to movement.

- If you play a song in your head—that is, if you only imagine it—you will naturally walk, and breathe, in time to its rhythm. (People in fearful or dangerous situations have survived by playing calming or fortifying music in their mind. Have you ever tried that? Did it work?)

- If you watch a dancer on the stage, your brain will respond to the rhythm that you hear and see, sending signals to your muscles, so that you (in some way) sense movement too. Moreover, there are studies that show that when we listen to a live music performance, as members of an audience, our brains collectively synchronize with the music and one another.

To move to rhythmic music is natural to us. Foot-tapping, so to speak, occurs at all levels of the nervous system. Hearing and responding to the beat actually makes us move—and helps us re-organize our movements if we're disabled in any way. Music therapy draws on that fact to develop rehabilitation protocols for people who have lost mobility, due to Parkinson's disease, stroke, traumatic brain injury, or other neurological disorders.

## What research and experience tells us: The example of Parkinson's disease

Over the years, clinicians have observed that auditory rhythm (the rhythm we hear)—drives motor function (the way we move). The implications for music therapy are significant. Put simply, **we may be able to manipulate rhythm to influence the way a person moves. This gives us a way to treat disorders of movement**, in people with Parkinson's disease, and people with hemiparesis (weakness or inability to move one side of the body) as a result of stroke or traumatic brain injury. Music interventions have been effective in treating these conditions for reasons that are only now emerging from neuroscience.

What we know is this: when sound enters the auditory system, it stimulates primary areas of motor function, such as the cerebellum, the motor cortex, and the basal ganglia. These are areas that are implicated in Parkinson's disease—and music gives us a way to reach them. An auditory pulse results in the actual stimulation of neurons in the basal ganglia, for example; so when someone listens to a musical rhythm, these neurons get *turned on*. In music therapy, this auditory pulse becomes a *rhythmic cue* that can have a therapeutic effect on movement.

### Music therapy for Parkinson's disease

People with Parkinson's disease have difficulties in moving, which show up as gait and balance problems, slowness of movement, inability to initiate movement (freezing and getting stuck), tremors, and uneven, erratic movements, among other symptoms. Auditory input from music, in the form of *rhythmic cues*, can stimulate the basal ganglia and other brain areas involved with motor timing. In particular, rhythmic cueing can influence the initiation of gait (walking) as well as the periodicity (regularity) of gait, including velocity and stride length, and the overall ease with which someone with Parkinson's disease can move. **Research shows that, over time, gait training with rhythmic cueing will result in measurable improvement in gait and balance for people with Parkinson's disease and other conditions that may impair gait, such as multiple sclerosis and stroke.**

But it's not a simple matter of providing an external beat for the person with Parkinson's disease: we need to provide *the right beat* for that person. Because Parkinson's disease affects the basal ganglia and other brain areas involved with motor timing, it also affects auditory *perception* of rhythm. There's been some research showing that people with Parkinson's disease may not hear or feel the beat where we think the beat should be. **So it's important to have a way of assessing which beat pattern works best for each patient,** and then use that pattern consistently.

Music therapists are trained to make this assessment, and to provide music to address rehabilitation goals. There's not enough funding for music therapists in rehabilitation settings, given the need. But here's the good news:

- Music therapy best practices are becoming part of rehabilitation, as a result of skill-sharing by music therapists.

- Technologies for gait training and other therapies based on rhythmic cueing, developed with input from music therapists, are becoming more widely available. (The music-enhanced treadmill, described below, is an example.) Physical therapists and occupational therapists are learning to apply these techniques to select music that has the desired beats per minute and rhythmic pattern for their patients with Parkinson's and other movement disorders.

*Example:*

An occupational therapist (who is not a musician) reports that he worked with a Parkinson's patient who was "shuffling" and did not respond well to "walking" music—maybe because it was too fast for him? The occupational therapist, who had had music therapy mentoring, experimented with different BPMs and identified a rate that worked for his patient. He created a list from Spotify of music that the patient could listen to through headphones, to therapeutic effect. The patient was "completely motivated," reported the occupational therapist, who was himself elated to discover that "you could choose music, from so many genres, for its impact on your patients." (Interview , D. Wilcox, OT, 5.05.22)

## TAKEAWAY
Exposure to music therapy best practices, and resources like Spotify, can empower members of the healthcare team to use music therapeutically in rehabilitation.

- During the Covid-19 pandemic, music therapists at the IMNF reached out to people with Parkinson's and their family care partners to provide virtual/hybrid programming. Below is a general description of an IMNF Parkinson's group that focuses on movement.

  - As a "check-in" before the first group session, participants with Parkinson's are assessed by the music therapist.

  - The music therapist then walks the care partner and person with Parkinson's through the process of finding the "right music," based on the initial assessment and the person's musical preferences. Each pair picks a "go-to song" for addressing ambulation issues. This can be done on the spot: the therapist identifies free services that will provide, for example, lists of 70s music at 80 BPM. Care partners learn how to use the go-to music (and other techniques) throughout the week, to reinforce benefits to patients. Other activities, such as drumming and chair exercises, may also be introduced in the zoom or hybrid sessions.

  Attendance in the groups (a key measure) and responses from participants have been very positive.

## TAKEAWAY
With assessment and oversight from a music therapist—and motivation from an online group—care partners and people with Parkinson's disease can learn to use music therapy best practices to support rehabilitation.

- Note that to be therapeutic for people with movement disorders, music therapy must respond to the needs of individual patients. And yet, music is often played in a rehabilitation gym, on the grounds that it will motivate and enhance the experience for patients generally. It is important to recognize that providing music in the rehabilitation gym is not music therapy—that is, it's not necessarily therapeutic for people with Parkinson's disease and movement disorders. The music provided may not provide the right beat, the right rhythmic cues, for individual patients—and may even be disruptive in some cases.

## Digital music technology: The musically enhanced treadmill

Gait training—which helps people walk better—is an important part of rehabilitation for people with Parkinson's disease. Physical therapists have used treadmills to provide forced gait training for stroke survivors and people with Parkinson's disease and multiple sclerosis, but it is only in recent years that a music-assisted treadmill has been developed with input from music therapists.

The Biodex Gait Trainer, for example, delivers music therapy-informed compositions that are specifically designed to support gait training for patients with varying needs and music preferences. The music therapist adjusts the tempo, dynamics, and other music components to the needs of the individual patient over the course of treatment. The Biodex musically enhanced treadmill provides real-time feedback to patients (which may be highly motivating), as well as print-outs of exercise outcome data for members of the healthcare team.

Clinical observations as well as controlled research studies have shown that most patients who use the musically enhanced treadmill show improvements in balance, stride length, symmetry, and velocity of gait—all of which carry over when they are out of therapy. Typically, as patients witness their improved function, their motivation increases and they participate more fully in their therapy sessions, leading to more rapid recovery. To observe a person with Parkinson's receiving Biodex music-assisted gait training, visit www.imnf.org/mhp-book-resources.

## Therapeutic dance for people with Parkinson's disease

Dance and other forms of rhythmic exercise promote wellness and enhance quality of life for just about everybody in senior care. It's clear that movement to music, informed by music therapy, can prevent falls, improve strength and balance, help focus attention, and kick-start the motivation for exercise among older people. Dance, in addition, offers a way of expressing oneself through the body, physically and emotionally, as part of a creative experience.

So it's not surprising that therapeutic dance has come to have a special role in helping people with Parkinson's disease.

A growing number of groups, in communities across the nation, provide dance for people with Parkinson's disease. These groups are led by therapists, professional dancers, and patients. Many kinds of dance are offered, including "PD-specific dance" (dance forms therapeutically designed for people with Parkinson's disease), modern dance, improvisational dance, American ballroom (waltz and foxtrot), and Argentine tango.

The tango, in particular, can be adapted to the needs of people with Parkinson's disease. Basically, the tango is a walking dance, requiring the dancer to step forward, and backward, and pivot in time to a strong rhythmic beat. The dance involves frequent stopping and starting of movement, as well as directional changes—all challenges for the person with Parkinson's disease. In fact, several tango step patterns seem to mimic the freezing of gait that occurs involuntarily in people with Parkinson's disease. These tango step patterns also mimic exercises that are prescribed as part of rehabilitation to help patients with Parkinson's disease achieve control of freezing of gait (Hackney & Earhart, 2009). In addition, the tango requires intimate rhythmic coordination with a partner, who (in many groups) is a volunteer experienced in the tango dance form and in the partnering of older dancers with rehabilitation goals. It seems to be a win-win for everybody.

## Dancing with Parkinson's: Pamela's story

Pamela G. Quinn is a professional dancer who has had Parkinson's disease for more than 20 years. When she received her diagnosis, at age 42, it was a devastating blow. "As a professional dancer, movement was my world," Quinn said, "it defined my identity, my income, my place." Quinn stopped taking dance class, stopped performing. And then she began to search for answers. But it turned out that her identity, if not her world, was still intact. She turned to her dance training to help her meet the daily challenges of Parkinson's disease. She began to develop—and then to invent—techniques for addressing the mobility issues she was experiencing. She created dances that explored her own experience, and went on to create group dances for others living with Parkinson's disease. She came to realize that she had much to give, as a dancer, teacher, innovator, and leader in the Parkinson's community.

In 2006, Quinn launched the PD Movement Lab in Brooklyn, New York, to explore new ways of helping people with Parkinson's disease through music, dance, imagery, and other strategies. Today the PD Movement Lab reaches classes throughout the US and Asia, and has a growing digital presence. Videos of Quinn's groups show people with Parkinson's disease working together to achieve greater mobility and physical freedom—and having fun as well.

In Quinn's words: "...equally important to challenging ourselves physically and mentally is the social experience of working, learning and playing together. We all need purpose, we all need movement, we all need connection."

Visit the PD Movement Lab at www.imnf.org/mhp-book-resources.

## Cognitive effects of therapeutic dance for people with movement disorders

Parkinson's disease is usually described as a movement disorder, characterized by physical symptoms, such as gait problems, freezing, and tremors. However, many people with Parkinson's experience cognitive impairments that affect daily function and quality of life. Cognitive impairments may show up as attention problems, slowness in remembering information, and difficulties in planning and carrying out tasks, for example. In some cases, a person with Parkinson's may develop more serious problems, including dementia.

Dance interventions have been shown to support cognitive health for older people; so it's not surprising that dance is therapeutic for people with Parkinson's disease who may be dealing with cognitive challenges. Consider that a person who participates in dance groups must learn (and then remember) dance steps, at first simple steps, and later more complex combinations. They will need to move, in time to the music, without confusing right foot with left, or right turn with left. They will need to navigate the dance space, with respect to other dancers who are moving through this space. These are, at some level, cognitive tasks. For people with Parkinson's disease, therapeutic dance may help protect against cognitive impairment associated with the disease.

Therapeutic dance is not always available in senior living facilities, or dance may be available in a limited way, in a recreational context. But what we are learning about therapeutic dance can influence the way we care for people with movement disorders.

## TAKEAWAYS

Here are some of the benefits of music/rhythmic interventions for people with Parkinson's disease:

- Moving to rhythmic music can be deeply helpful to people

with Parkinson's disease and other movement disorders, who have lost some of their "inner music."

- Rhythmic cues help people move in time to the music. Rhythmic cues from an external source, such as a recording or musically enhanced treadmill, are used by music therapists, physical therapists, and occupational therapists to help people with Parkinson's disease regulate their gait, improve posture and balance, and regain fluidity in their movements.

- By rhythmic cues we usually mean an auditory pulse or beat. But, especially in therapeutic dance, rhythmic cues can also be visual or social—for example, cues that come to patients from *other people who are moving, dancing, or playing music along with them*. Rhythmic cues make people move together. This is because there is a natural tendency to get in sync with the rhythms around us, not just musical rhythms, but all kinds of rhythms. For example, we tend to adjust our walking rhythm to the rhythm of a person who is walking in front of us. And when we are doing repetitive physical work, we tend to get in rhythm with others on our team: if you and the kids are chopping vegetables in the kitchen, it won't be long before you are chopping in unison. This tendency for our responses to fall into rhythm with an external signal is an example of the phenomenon of entrainment, discussed earlier. It's easy to see how entrainment helps people walk together or work together—and why a person with Parkinson's might choose to walk behind a stranger in the street as a way of regularizing their gait.

Experience shows that people with Parkinson's disease respond well to therapies that are strongly based in rhythmic cueing, such as gait training on a musically enhanced treadmill, or participating in therapeutic dance. In addition, many people with Parkinson's disease benefit from music therapy techniques that are used in rehabilitation of patients with stroke, traumatic brain injury, amputation, and other movement disorders. These therapies are discussed below.

## Stroke: An introduction

In the US, stroke is a leading cause of serious long-term disability. Every year, nearly 800,000 people in the US have a stroke, and for most (about 75%) this is a first stroke. African-Americans and Hispanic Americans are disproportionately represented among stroke victims—and this is one of many glaring health disparities that ought to concern us as a nation (Centers for Disease Control and Prevention, n.d.). A stroke occurs when something blocks blood supply to part of the brain, or when a blood vessel in the brain bursts, damaging nearby brain tissue. The CDC tells us that a stroke is sometimes called a "brain attack." A medical term for stroke is CVA or cerebrovascular accident, which tells us that the attack involves both the brain (denoted by "cerebro") and the blood vessels (or "vascular" system).

The words "accident" and "attack" capture an important reality. Stroke is an injury or insult to the brain, sudden and often unexpected. It is also a medical emergency. This is because blood carries oxygen to the brain, as to all other parts of the body, and when something happens to disrupt the normal flow of blood to the brain, brain cells are starved of oxygen and begin to die within minutes. If not treated immediately, a stroke can cause permanent brain damage and long-term disability, or even death. (Treatment involves quick action to remove or dissolve a blood clot that is blocking blood supply, or to stop the bleeding from a burst vessel.)

For the patient and their family, the stroke begins as an emergency, which may be followed by a long period of neurological recovery and rehabilitation.

The nature and severity of stoke disability varies, depending on the area of the brain that is affected, and the extent of the damage. More than half of stroke survivors aged 65 or over experience problems in mobility. If the stroke (the accident) has occurred in the right hemisphere of the brain, then the left side of the body will be affected, and vice versa. Likely effects are weakness, loss of feeling, or even paralysis on the affected side. The stroke survivor may need to re-learn how to stand or walk, or to move an arm and hand to grasp or hold objects, again on the affected side. Speech may also be affected. Brain areas affecting speech are found mostly in the left hemispheres, so patients with left-hemisphere damage may need to re-learn how to speak, or process and understand language, again depending on the specific area affected.

In sum, a stroke is most likely to cause one or more of these disabilities:

- Movement problems

- Problems in using and/or understanding language

- Sensory problems:

- Pain

- Problems with proprioception (not knowing where one's body is; not being able to move freely and safely in the environment)

- "Visual neglect" (or "spatial neglect"): an inability to pay attention to, process, or "see" one side of the environment—most often the left side, due to damage to the visual or sensory areas of the right hemisphere of the brain

• Problems with thinking and memory

• Emotional challenges.

Because stroke survivors often experience serious long-term disabilities, they are well represented in long-term care facilities. As we have learned to treat stroke disabilities more effectively, stroke survivors are also successfully treated in the short-term subacute rehabilitation units of senior care facilities, and through home-delivered services.

Recent advances in neuroscience have shown that there is a greater capacity for neurologic recovery from stroke than was previously acknowledged. For example, clinical research in music therapy has identified music interventions that are uniquely effective in addressing mobility and speech problems—as well as the psychological challenges that are part of being a stroke survivor.

## Music therapy and stroke
### Beginning where the person is

In neurological rehabilitation, the first thing that needs our attention is the experience of the person before us. This is especially true when that person has experienced a traumatic event, such as a stroke or amputation.

Michael H. Thaut, PhD, a research leader in the neuroscience of music and its applications to rehabilitation, refers to the "shaken sense of self" that is experienced by stroke victims. He writes:

> The first issue that needs attention in neurological rehabilitation is the person's disrupted identity. After a neurological injury or illness with its accompanying cognitive losses, the following questions may emerge: *Who am I? Why am I different? Why can't I do the things I did before? Why do people treat me differently? What will happen to me? Will I regain my former abilities? Effective cognitive rehabilitation needs to help the person establish a sense of self in a way that assists him or her in achieving stability.* (Thaut, 2005, p.182)

In other words, the first step in engaging a patient in rehabilitation is to consider the patient's subjective experience—how the patient feels and thinks about themselves. To do this we will need to identify—and address—the patient's immediate emotional and cognitive needs, the "shaken sense of self." Module 4 explores music interventions that help people cope with isolation, depression symptoms, and other emotional challenges that may be experienced by stroke survivors.

## Movement rehabilitation for stroke: Using a person's connection to music to drive physical movement

As we have seen, music therapy for people with Parkinson's disease includes gait training, which uses rhythmic cues from recorded music. Some stroke patients who have difficulty walking may also benefit from gait training. Gait training can also help people who have had a traumatic brain injury (TBI), such as a concussion or head injury: and that's because TBI often shows up as difficulties in walking, or moving forward in a healthy, rhythmic way. Some stroke and TBI patients will make good use of the musically enhanced treadmill or other forms of rhythmic cueing—but, as with Parkinson's patients, their options don't end there.

## Music patterns as cues for movement

The music that is used for therapeutic purposes brings into play not just rhythm, but also other elements of music—including pitch, tempo, loudness, and timbre (reflecting the sound quality of different instruments). All of these elements come together to create the sound patterns that we hear as music. For example, sounds with different pitches come together to create the music patterns we call melody and harmony. It is the overarching music patterns that we respond to in our favorite songs, in dance music, and—significantly— in exercise music too. Music with a soaring melody, or music that is loud, fast, and dissonant, moves us in a different way from music that is steady, gentle, and of moderate pace.

**Music therapists are trained to identify music patterns that will help individual patients with stroke or brain injuries to move in ways that are therapeutic for them.** For example, a stroke survivor may benefit from exercises to maintain movement in an arm or leg affected by the stroke, and gradually improve range of motion. The music therapist will select or improvise music in which the music pattern exactly fits the needs of the person who is undergoing rehabilitation. The goal is to build up a repertoire of exercises to help stroke survivors practice the movements that they will need in order to function, as well as possible, in daily life.

Here are some examples showing why it works:

- **Melodies** move forward in time, and also in auditory space, and as the arc of a melody moves up or down, it engages us to move as well.

  - An expansive and mostly ascending melodic line can lift up a patient, *physically* and *emotionally*, in the moment. The music therapist will offer a melody that is ascending as a cue to movement. As the patient listens to the ascending melody, attuned to movement or dance, she may feel like reaching upward, breathing upward, and perhaps thinking upward too. Familiar melodies can keep the patient fully engaged for the duration of a song, not only enhancing movement but endurance.

    What about melodic lines that are mostly descending? As you might expect, an expansive, mostly descending melody may cue downward movement. But this same melody may deliver a physical pick-me-up as well: as we listen to a descending melody, we *actively expect* the melody to again reach upward; and (except, possibly, at the end of the piece) it always does. So we do too! Descending melodies have the potential to deliver physical release, or the emotional release that we call catharsis.

    Expansive melodies can help patients move to music in a way that expands their reach and range of motion. Moving (or just listening to) an expansive melody may generate energy and defuse depression as well. For examples of ascending and descending melodies, visit www.imnf.org/mhp-book-resources.

  - When a melody is not expansive, but hovers around a central tonal point, this may support smaller, more focused movements. The famous "Ode to Joy" by Beethoven is not an expansive melody; it uses no more than five connecting tones, within the scope of one hand (with only one punctuating exception). But it builds a physical and emotional response by other means—its intensity, for example: achieved by a strong pulse (as opposed to a free-flowing rhythm).

    The point is that the melody is a cue for movement, and music therapists choose melodies that help individual patients with stroke or brain injuries move in ways that are therapeutic for them.

- **Dynamics**, or loudness/softness in music, can also drive movement for a stroke patient. Increasing loudness can drive a gradual movement toward expansion (a patient reaching outward, rhythmically, with larger movements), and softening can cue smaller and more centered movements.

- **Harmony**, which includes tone clusters in either open or closed positions, can also "cue" or stimulate large or small movements, as well as the emotional responses that drive movement that is potentially therapeutic. Harmonic clusters can sound bright and energizing to further encourage active participation.

Music therapy for stroke and TBI survivors should be overseen by music therapists who have established a therapeutic relationship with their patient. Knowing the patient's relationship with music is important, as this will affect how fully the patient can engage in the experience and benefit from music-based interventions. The music therapist needs to integrate all of the patient's music listening and music-making experiences into the rehabilitation plan.

To understand how music patterns affect movement, try a simple experiment—moving to chords (with notes played together) versus arpeggios (the same notes played one after another). Access this experiment at www.imnf. org/mhp-book-resources.

## Music-making and singing in support of rehabilitation

Playing a musical instrument or singing a song involves movement—and that movement may be directed toward rehabilitation goals.

For a stroke survivor, the music therapist may select a musical instrument that requires participation of the stroke-affected arm, a little at first, then at increasingly manageable levels. Making music helps the patient initiate and practice movements that have therapeutic value. And for patients with very limited movement, adaptive instruments, which are finely tuned to the patient's physical abilities, are used in rehabilitation (see below).

Singing and chanting require no instruments other than the human voice. For patients with pain and low motivation, the music therapist or family care partner can often find a song with a refrain that can be sung or chanted to help the person push through the pain and find the strength and confidence to persevere through a demanding rehabilitation program.

**For patients with movement disorders, singing or playing a musical instrument has the potential to improve function, reduce pain, strengthen motivation, and put recovery in reach. In some cases, the music-making offers a chance for self-expression, including expression of the anger or frustration that is often involved in rehabilitation after a stroke or injury.**

**Singing through pain**

For facilities that provide short-term rehabilitation, music-making can be an important part of the care plan. Here is the first of two examples of how singing can help support the rehabilitation process:

> *Example:* Mary was a patient in our facility for short-term rehabilitation fol-lowing a stroke that left her with muscle weakness, and balance and mobility issues. Due to severe pain, she was using a wheelchair. She had difficulty getting up from the chair and could only take a few steps before giving up. The music therapist worked with Mary to find a song with a good rhythm that she found inspiring. The music therapist told Mary to sing this while she was trying to step up and out of her wheelchair. As Mary started to sing "If I can just...hold...out til tomor...row, If I can just...keep...faith...through the night. If I can just...hold...out til tomorrow...everything...will...be al...right." Singing this in a slow deliberate tempo, Mary not only walked a few steps but walked the full length of the unit without stopping or sitting in her chair to rest. The song carried her and she was able to use it consistently to walk independently again. The song also had a message of hope and motivated her to "hold out" and not give up.

For some patients, physical therapy seems too painful and they give up. Low motivation or depression prevents them from taking the first steps toward the recovery that is possible. Music interventions can help restore mood, motivation, and the inner rhythm that is involved in caring about oneself.

> *Example:* Linda was a young adult in a skilled nursing facility following a severe injury resulting from a car accident. She was extremely discouraged and couldn't motivate herself to ask to be taken out of bed to go to rehab. Physical therapy was too painful, so she tried to avoid it. The music therapist was asked to visit her in her room. The music therapist started with a breath-ing exercise, asking Linda to take a deep breath in, and to breathe out on a sung long sigh "aah," and to feel the vibration in her chest and back as she sighed out. During this, the music therapist played sustained chords on the keyboard to support and amplify the resonance of Linda's sigh. Linda found these toned breathing exercises comforting. Using the same tone of Linda's sigh, the music therapist chanted "I am strong" and then asked Linda to do the same. The music therapist then asked Linda for a song that would give her the feeling of strength. Linda chose Gloria Gaynor's "I Will Survive." With its disco beats and inspirational message, the song gave Linda strength, and she was encouraged to keep a recording of the song with her, to motivate her to get out of bed and go to her rehab therapy sessions. With this, her physical therapy could begin in earnest.

Note that in this example, the music therapist offered breathing exercises, supported by music that responded, in the moment, to the emotional needs of a person facing rehabilitation. Music therapists are trained in techniques that help patients like Linda. But caregivers without any special training can help a patient or loved one find a "go-to song" that they find inspirational and motivating—and therefore therapeutic.

Here are some tips for using songs to support rehabilitation:

- Generally, the go-to song for rehabilitation will have a regular rhythm that drives or motivates movement, as well as an inspirational message and *personal meaning*.

- The song can be short and contain improvised phrases such as "I am strong," "I can do this," "I will hold on" ("Hold on Mary, hold on"). In other words, you don't need the whole song, or the "right" words. The content for this phrase needs to come from the person who is the patient. A music therapist can bring this together. But if you are a family caregiver or an experienced caregiver, you too are in a good position to help your loved one or patient find the right song and the right words.

- Typically, the song that is used for motivation (a "get-out-of-bed song") will be upbeat and played at a driving tempo. A song that is used to support step-by-step rehabilitation may be altered or improvised in response to the patient's movement, in the moment (as described in the example of Mary singing through pain).

Caregivers and family care partners can help their patients or loved ones use music interventions, such as singing, to get the most out of short-term rehabilitation—to let the music carry them, past pain and depression, so that they can hope for and fully participate in their recovery.

## Music-making with adaptive musical instruments

Playing a musical instrument is therapeutic on many levels, and that's why music therapists use a dazzling array of instruments to help people with depression, dementia, stroke, and other health challenges. For people who have had a stroke or injury, playing a musical instrument is a form of movement therapy, similar in its goals to occupational therapy: it is an activity that is task-oriented, with the potential to improve motor skills. Music therapists use musical instruments that require a person to perform specific movements in order to create sound. The person's efforts to play the instrument are designed to bring about desired outcomes, such as improved fine motor coordination, strength, flexibility, and range of motion.

The use of musical instruments in stroke rehabilitation motivates patients by offering them enjoyable and creative music experiences that accelerate the rehabilitation process. At the same time, music-making gives patients a chance to express their feelings, including feelings of frustration, by creating sounds that are powerful and expressive (Paul & Ramsey, 2000).

## How it works

The healthcare team, including the physical therapist and occupational therapist, identifies the rehabilitation goals for the patient, and, with the music therapist, determines whether or not the patient is likely to benefit from music therapy.

We should note that although the notion of "rehabilitation" is strongly associated with "improvement," music therapy may be indicated for stroke, TBI, and amputation survivors who appear to have reached their maximum level of functioning. For some patients, music therapy results in improvements that could not be achieved through physical therapy or occupational therapy alone. For other patients, music therapy may help *maintain* maximum level of functioning, which might otherwise decline.

- **The patient does not need to have had music training, or to have played a musical instrument, to participate in therapeutic music-making. An interest in music, or an inclination to listen to music, is all that is required.**

- As a first step, the music therapist learns about the music identity of the patient—which styles of music the patient prefers, and what music experiences have been most meaningful to them. For example has the patient sung in a community choir? Did they take piano lessons as a child? Have they always wanted to play the guitar? With this background, the music therapist matches the patient to a specific instrument that reflects their interests and can be adapted to their physical abilities.

  - Musical instruments include keyboards, xylophones, guitars, violins, flutes, and so on, as well as many simple percussive instruments, such as drums, tambourines, jingle bells, shakers, tone bars, and frame drums.

- **For patients with very limited physical abilities, music therapists offer specialized instruments, adapted to respond to the patient's available movement with a full and pleasing sound.**

– Music therapists may adapt a conventional instrument, for example adding a built-up handle to a drumstick, so that it can be used by a person with a weak handgrip (Paul & Ramsey, 2000). Also available are electronic musical instruments and devices that can be programmed to enable people with very limited movements to produce sound.

*Example:* Music therapists helped Willie, a TBI patient, to access a keyboard through a pointer stick worn over his head like a baseball cap. Because Willie was seriously impaired, getting him to interact with a music keyboard synthesizer required some adaptations. Physically, the layout of the piano keys was longer than Willie's range of motion. To compensate for this, the keyboard was reconfigured: pitches associated with the middle register of the keyboard were digitally remapped to the upper register, so that Willie could reach them. Willie began to pick out songs, and after a few weeks he felt like he was "born to do this."…"It's really different that something comes so easily to me," he said, when everything else had been a real struggle (Nagler, 1998).

- It is important to take into account the emotional state of the patient. Often, people who have suffered a stroke or other injury will begin rehabilitation with a "shaken sense of self." They may resist playing a musical instrument, due to depression or fear of failure in a new activity. They may protest that they are "not musical." The music therapist may begin by talking with the patient, playing familiar music, and improvising in response to the patient's needs. In a group setting, the patient will also be encouraged by the participation of other members.

- In an individual session, the music therapist and patient will play music together; in a group session, the therapist will work with three to four patients. Sessions are designed to help each group member express themselves musically on their chosen instrument. This will require that group members initiate movement in parts of the body that have limited movement. With continued playing, members may improve fine motor skills, hand-eye coordination, and other motor skills that are important to daily activities.

  Playing an instrument in a group will also require that the members learn to coordinate with others through music and movement. Listening and paying attention to cues in the music-making session may improve visual and auditory perception.

- Playing a musical instrument has psychological benefits for people in movement rehabilitation, as for other patients. The focus of the music-making is to create a real product (the music). Achieving this enhances a person's self-esteem, and brings pleasure to other participants.

- Playing a musical instrument also gives a person the chance to master a new ability, or to revisit an activity that has given pleasure in the past. For some people, music-making on a chosen instrument is part of their identity, and this presents special opportunities, as well as challenges, to rehabilitation. Music therapists have developed many ways to help people who are amateur or professional musicians to compensate for physical losses. For example, a stroke survivor who has limited movement on one side of their body may continue to play the piano, fully, and to their own satisfaction, with one hand. (There is, in fact, a substantial repertoire for piano performance using one hand only.) Adaptations for other instruments can help lifelong musicians use music in rehabilitation.

## Specialized electronic music-making devices— piezo triggers and much more

More than 25 years ago, IMNF music therapists began to pioneer the use of specialized electronic instruments in movement rehabilitation. Music and recreational therapists were eager to use drumming in rehabilitation—because it engaged patients in a very positive way. But music therapists noticed that some physically impaired patients could not sound a drum: they lacked the fine motor skills to disengage from the head of a drum once struck, and this prevented the drum from resonating. To work around this, music therapists began affixing electronic triggers (called *piezo triggers*) to the back of drum surfaces. The triggers convert stimuli into musical instrument digital information (MIDI), a computer language that is sent to a converter to produce sound. With the added sensitivity of MIDI (which we can program), a person can activate musical sounds with the slightest touch. The arrival of MIDI-based instruments was truly game-changing for therapists and patients engaged in rehabilitation.

Piezo triggers are among the simplest of a whole class of adaptive instruments that use MIDI interfaces. What all of these instruments have in common is that they allow a person with limited movement to create sounds from a digital sound module. These sounds can be of any instrument type the person chooses: drums, piano, guitar, flute—the possibilities are endless! **There are music-based apps and a new array of switches that can be used to help almost everyone engage in musical expression regardless of**

**their physical limitations.** Laptop and desktop computers, portable keyboards with built-in speakers, phones and tablets, and other devices can run software that can create music over a speaker, and through connections or interfaces with other devices.

For people who have suffered a stroke, brain injury, or amputation, access to adaptive music technology can have powerful benefits. In our simple piezo trigger example, occupational therapy issues can be addressed through music-making, since the activity of drumming (striking and releasing) involves fine motor coordination, a range of motion, and a certain level of muscle strength. What's more, with this kind of computer-monitored music-making, progress can be measured, providing direct feedback to the patient and healthcare team, to guide therapy.

Music-making offers many therapeutic options for stroke survivors and for others who have limited movement as a result of TBI or other injuries. Using the adaptive instrument, the person moves their body in a way that creates the response they want, in the form of sound, and music. In so doing they achieve a kind of control over their environment, and are, at the same time, able to express their feelings.

(More information on emerging music technology and its uses in music therapy appears in our discussion of "Technology and Virtual Programming: Expanding Access to Music Therapy and Music Programming", toward the end of the book, and in a review of current and emergent technology available at www.imnf.org/mhp-book-resources.)

### "I am a musician"

The mastery of the adaptive instrument increases a person's self-esteem, and often the motivation to succeed in rehabilitation and other areas of life. For people who are, or who feel as if they are, seriously disabled, music-making is a chance to define themselves as someone other than "the patient." The identity is now "I am a musician." And—here's the beauty of it—if music-making is recorded, computer software makes it possible for the music therapist or a technician to edit the music created during the session to a high standard, to be valued and shared with others.

## "We are musicians": The voices of IMNF patients who have used adaptive music instruments in rehabilitation

### Robert

Robert had struggled with polio and other lifelong physical handicaps. When he came to long-term care, he didn't want to go to physical therapy or take any part in his rehabilitation. He was referred to music therapy, where electronic instruments and production capabilities were available to him. The music therapist soon learned that Robert had written several songs more than 35 years ago, while he was living in Las Vegas. The swing styles of Sammy Davis Jr. and Frank Sinatra came through in these compositions. After the second music therapy session, he and his music therapist recorded his first song, "Crazy Little World."

In producing this song, Robert was able to make something that reminded him of his healthy creative self. And he was able to share that self with his music therapist, and later with others. Robert told his music therapist, "This motivates me to do more with my life. I'm even showing up to physical therapy on time."

## Lil

Lil never had any music training. Severely disabled by cerebral palsy, she came to a music-making group because she loved music and really enjoys socializing. The tambourine became her favorite instrument. She was able to play it with her foot.

Every once in a while, Lil came to the group crying, and saying, "I'm disabled, I'm disabled!" (Well so are we all, the group might say—but that is not what they said.) The group members, led by a music therapist, understood that Lil needed something extra now and then, and they composed a song, "Here Comes Lil," to remind her that she was loved and valued. And this song, this music, served to reconnect her to her social and creative self, so that she could put her foot to the tambourine once again.

## Kevin

Kevin never learned to play a musical instrument, despite having been involved in music technology for many years. He composed songs, but they remained in his highly developed musical memory, and were not realized in the world of others. Kevin had been living with Parkinson's disease for many years and had serious cognitive and physical limitations. He began working with a music therapy intern who was receiving special training in music technology as part of a special program. Kevin was able to record his compositions. In the recordings, the therapist captured difficult melodic lines and arranged jazz harmonies that reflected Kevin's creative intentions. His music, Kevin says, is truly a dream that came true.

## Music therapy for "visual (or spatial) neglect"

Stroke not only affects those areas of the brain that control movement and language; in some cases, damage to the sensory and visual areas of the brain creates a phenomenon called visual or spatial neglect, or "hemineglect" (for left hemisphere neglect). In visual neglect, damage to the right hemisphere results in a person's inability to attend to, process, or "see" things that appear in the left side of their visual environment.

In severe cases of visual neglect, the patients behave as if objects to their left side aren't there; even parts of their own body, a left leg for example, seem not to be within their view or attention. In less severe cases, only the periphery of the visual space may be affected.

Visual neglect is a brain problem, not a vision problem. And because the brain's auditory centers may remain intact, music therapists are often able to restore the patient's awareness of the left side of the environment through auditory stimuli, including music. For example, a patient with visual neglect may not "see" or process the existence of a glass of water that is placed to their left. But if we position a sound-making instrument, such as a set of handbells, so that it extends into the neglected left field, we can guide the patient to play the bells, from right to left. Since there is no damage to their auditory awareness, they will hear the bells to the left; which will guide them to become aware of the bells, and thus to recognize, and focus on, other stimuli in the neglected area. Through such interventions, patients with visual neglect can begin to fill in the missing half of their visual field, which in turn will help them manage activities of daily life. To watch a music therapy intervention for visual neglect, visit www.imnf.org/mhp-book-resources.

# MODULE 8

# Music Therapy and Speech Rehabilitation

Speech, or the ability to communicate through some form of language, is said to be unique to humans—maybe, even, "what makes us human." Certainly this is true if we are referring to the ability to communicate complex thoughts and ideas through words, sounds, or symbols.

Consider this: in no other species has the brain evolved to support language that is as advanced as that of an ordinary human child in the second year of life. Only machines, created by humans, can speak, understand, and respond as well as we do (or almost as well). The human brain is primed to develop languages (including computer languages and other languages in our future): it's what we do.

The language that is part of our genetic heritage includes not only speech, but an array of abilities that make it possible for us to communicate with one another. These abilities include:

- Receptive abilities:

    - Listening to and understanding the speech of other people.

    - Reading, or receiving word/symbolic communications in some other way that facilitates communication.

- Expressive abilities:

    - Speaking to other people, with words, as well as vocal cues and physical gestures.

    - Writing, or expressing oneself to others in words or some other symbolic way (e.g. through images or pictorials that can be translated into "language").

Different brain areas work together, rhythmically, to support each of these behaviors. Most important are the "language areas" of the brain that account for our ability to turn thoughts into words, and to speak and understand language. *But other areas of the brain are involved as well.* For example, listening involves hearing; reading involves sight. Sensory areas of the brain and nervous system are involved in these and other language behaviors. Speaking requires that we use our mouths, tongues, lips, and all the muscles of our face; writing requires a fine coordination of the hands; and so motor areas of the brain are also involved.

**Because language behavior is so complex, a lot of backup is built into the system. That is, the brain allows for many different pathways to language.**

## Language disorders

Language abilities begin to develop in earliest childhood, with babbling, then first words, then sentences, and the exponential growth of vocabulary and comprehension as the brain matures. In some cases, though, over the course of a lifetime, the language areas of the brain are damaged by illness or injury, resulting in language disorders. As we age, sensory losses are also common— not hearing well, for example. In fact, many of the challenges experienced by older people involve some loss of language or communication abilities.

In senior care and rehabilitation settings, the most serious language losses are seen among people with dementia, and among stroke survivors. People with dementia gradually lose the ability to speak or understand speech, as the language areas of the brain are devastated over the course of this progressive brain disease. People who have survived a stroke or TBI (traumatic brain injury) may lose certain language abilities, depending on the location and extent of the brain damage they have experienced.

*Aphasia* is the general term for language disorders that result from direct damage to one or more language areas of the brain—as happens in stroke and TBI. One of the most common types of aphasia is *expressive aphasia*, in which a person is unable to speak ("express") more than a few words (or maybe none at all), but is able to understand the speech of others. Music therapy is well recognized as an effective treatment for people with expressive aphasia (also called Broca's aphasia, and non-fluent aphasia).

## Music as a pathway to language (and memory, and movement, and more)

More than 40 years ago, clinicians in long-term care settings began to notice that music had an almost magical effect on some of their patients. That is, there was something about music—the auditory system and its connections— that could restore function to those with severe neurologic impairments.

- For example, music therapists discovered that music could reach people with late-stage Alzheimer's disease, when nothing else did. There were patients who were unable to talk, and sometimes unable to remember the names of their children. And yet when a music therapist engaged them with a familiar song, they responded by singing—finding, or remembering, the words of the song.

- We discovered that music could help people with Parkinson's disease. When music therapists prescribed rhythmic music as part of rehabilitation, patients who had been unable to move without halting or freezing were able to walk, or even dance, again.

- And just as remarkable, we discovered that many stroke survivors who were unable to speak could sing or hum familiar songs. We saw patients who struggled to say a word or two, in a flat or toneless manner, but were able to sing snatches of songs expressively, without apparent effort.

In each of these clinical examples, the "almost magic" effect of music is, in fact, grounded in neurophysiology or brain function.

**TAKEAWAY**
When brain damage results in a loss of function through normal neurological pathways, music may be able to provide an alternative pathway—to memory, to movement, and to language and speech.

We begin with our discussion of music therapy for aphasia, with an introduction by Oliver Sacks, MD, at www.imnf.org/mhp-book-resources.

## Music therapy for aphasia: Why it works (when it works)
Based on clinical observations, music therapists hypothesized that music and singing might be a pathway to speech rehabilitation for some of their stroke and TBI patients. And this has proven to be so.

Patients with aphasia typically have incurred damage to the left hemisphere of the brain. But music processing in the right hemisphere is not affected. For some patients with aphasia, the brain systems that respond to music have the potential to support language as well. Here's why:

- There is no one "music area" in the brain. Instead, there are numerous brain systems that respond to particular musical experience and skills, and these are distributed throughout the brain.

- The areas involved in language processing, by contrast, are mostly located in definable areas of the brain: in the left hemisphere for people who are right-handed, and for about half of those who are left-handed as well. This means that a stroke that damages the speech areas on the left side of the brain will likely result in language losses. What then?

## Brain plasticity

**The brain has the ability to make new neural connections, to re-wire itself, so to speak, as it responds to experiences of all kinds. This ability is called** *brain plasticity.* ("Plasticity" here means the exact opposite of "fixed"—that is, flexible, or malleable.)

Brain plasticity is part of your life, whatever you do. For example, if you learn to play the flute, ride a bicycle, or read braille with your fingertips, your brain will develop neural connections that reflect and enable these activities. We can see from brain imaging that there are characteristic differences between the brains of lifelong musicians and non-musicians, between flutists and drummers, and so forth. Among the musicians, the parts of the brain involved in music processing, and in the movements required to play their particular instrument, appear larger, with greater connectivity. Playing your instrument changes your brain over time (as does riding a bicycle and much else that you learn to do).

**Brain plasticity is not only the basis for learning and adaptation throughout life; it also helps us to recover from brain injuries.** If a language function, such as speech production, has been compromised by brain damage, the brain can adapt by finding an alternate pathway to achieve that function. Music often provides this alternate pathway. And when function improves, there is always a network change that accompanies this improvement, and makes further improvement possible.

In the early days of brain research, language and music were assumed to be independent brain functions. **But recent cognitive research and brain-imaging suggests that language and music are processed in similar ways in the brain, which means that they can sometimes share brain resources.** For example, both language and music rely on syntax, in that words (or tones) are arranged in a certain order, for meaning or effect. The brain knows how to process syntax—in language and in music. And it uses similar processing to decode a sentence or a tune. So there is overlap between the processing of language and music.

The overlap between music and language processing provides a kind of "backup" for people with aphasia. As noted, these patients have typically incurred damage to the left hemisphere of the brain. But music processing in the right hemisphere is not affected.

This means that if a person experiences a stroke or TBI that takes out one or more language areas of the brain, the brain may recruit complementary or parallel networks from the right hemisphere to compensate for lost language function, in whole or part. Sometimes a person recovers language functions in the first six months after a stroke or injury. If not, adaptation takes time, and requires the coordinated efforts of the stroke survivor and the rehabilitation team. Music therapy helps initiate and ground this process.

## Expressive aphasia (also called non-fluent aphasia or Broca's aphasia)

Before the arrival of brain imaging, physicians were dependent on autopsies that might (or might not) validate their hypotheses about what was causing the neurological problems of their patients. In 1861, a French physician, Paul Broca, discovered, on autopsy, that a patient who was unable to speak had suffered damage to an area of the frontal lobe, in the left hemisphere. He concluded that this area was responsible for speech production. Broca's discovery was validated by clinical observations, and later by brain science: damage to this brain area, now known as Broca's area, results in loss of speech, or expressive aphasia.

The term expressive *aphasia* recognizes that the disorder affects expression or production of speech (as opposed to the ability to receive speech). That is, people with expressive aphasia have difficulty speaking, but are able to understand the speech of others. Other names for the disorder are Broca's aphasia, and non-fluent aphasia. The descriptive term "non-fluent" recognizes that a defining characteristic of this disorder is the inability to produce fluent or free-flowing speech. A person with expressive or non-fluent aphasia may be able to say a few words or phrases. But the melody and the rhythm of ordinary speech is lost; there are irregular pauses, as the person struggles to find the word; sentences may consist of mainly nouns and verbs, without the connective words and phrases.

### Treating expressive aphasia

Patients who are diagnosed with expressive or non-fluent aphasia are assessed by a speech-language pathologist using a variety of standardized assessment tools (such as the Boston Aphasia Battery). Speech therapy begins as soon as possible, as progress is most likely to occur in the first weeks after the stroke or injury.

### Speech therapy

Speech therapy for expressive or non-fluent aphasia typically involves structured exercises in which the patient repeats and rehearses phrases, practices
naming objects presented in pictures, and practices reading out loud. Patients
will also listen to recordings of themselves, as feedback and instruction. They
may use computer-based programs to rehearse standard phrases and practice
skills in between therapy sessions.

For people with expressive aphasia, speech therapy is intensive and often
exhausting. At the outset, there may be few opportunities to feel successful,
so motivation is often a challenge. Many patients progress to the point where
they are able to initiate phrases and sentences. But often patients reach a
plateau after six months and, under managed care guidelines, are discontinued for treatment. Research indicates that intensive treatment in the weeks
following a stroke or TBI has better outcomes than fewer hours per week
over a longer period of time.

Music therapy may be added at any point in treatment. For patients who
have been unable to reach their goals through speech therapy alone, music
therapy is often successful. Patients referred for music therapy for expressive
aphasia are first assessed for cognitive function, to ensure that they are able
to understand instructions and process information. No music background
or training is necessary.

## Music therapy approaches to expressive aphasia: An introduction

Music therapy for people with expressive aphasia uses musical vocalization, in
its many forms, to retrain people to speak. Below is an overview of the major
music therapy approaches to aphasia. The actual music therapy plan for a
survivor of stroke or TBI will be more comprehensive, including techniques
that address individual needs around breathing, vocal quality, articulation,
word retrieval ability, and more.

Music therapy for speech rehabilitation will be carried out by a music
therapist in partnership with a speech-language pathologist. Some music
therapy techniques can also be learned and reinforced by caregiving staff and
family care partners. And it helps if the person with aphasia, and everyone
involved in their care, understands what music can contribute to recovery.
We've highlighted the basics here.

### Singing familiar songs

Beginning a treatment session with familiar songs helps create a therapeutic
environment that is enjoyable and engaging. The patient is asked to select

a song that is familiar and enjoyable—for example, "You Are My Sunshine," "This Little Light of Mine." Together, therapist and patient focus on the most familiar parts of the song, repeating them, as in a refrain. Tempo and dynamics are adjusted to take into account what the patient can do, physically, in the aftermath of a stroke or TBI, and what they want to do, at the expressive level. A therapeutic interaction is established between the music therapist through engagement with the song and its expression.

Note that in treating people with aphasia, music therapists do not favor songs that elicit memories or emotional responses; they choose songs that are familiar, enjoyable, and, for most people, easy to sing. A strong emotional response to the song would distract from the hard work of speech rehabilitation; moreover, the person with aphasia would have no way of processing their feelings through discussion. You can see why the role of familiar songs in aphasia treatment would be different from their role in the treatment of people with dementia, depression symptoms, and other mental health challenges.

The advantage of beginning music-based aphasia therapy with familiar songs is that it has a greater than average chance of success. **Singing bypasses the impaired language centers in the left hemisphere, allowing some people with aphasia to sing words and phrases, when speech seems almost impossible.**

**As therapy progresses, the music therapist uses musical cues to encourage more interaction and emotional expression.** For example, the therapist may vary the song flow, and pause at the last words of each phrase of the song—at which point the patient will complete the phrase, with pleasure in the music, and growing confidence in their recovery.

## Musically assisted speech

At the beginning of treatment, people with expressive aphasia differ greatly in their ability to sing words and phrases from familiar songs. No one size— no one treatment—fits all. What music therapy-based approaches have in common is that they are designed to help people with aphasia regain their ability to communicate by first singing words and phrases—as opposed to simply speaking them.

*Musically assisted speech* is a general term for treatment in which conversational phrases are embedded in melodic phrases to support speech. The music therapist begins with simple, basic communications. If the patient has good comprehension, the music therapist identifies phrases of use, and sets these phrases to familiar music. (For example, the greeting "Hello, how are you today?" can be set to the tune of "Swing Low, Sweet Chariot;" "It's good to see you" can be set to "Happy Birthday to You.") For some patients, phrases will be shorter, two or three syllables/musical tones; for example, "I'm okay" can be paired with "Three Blind Mice." These musically assisted phrases will be practiced in the music therapy sessions, and played out in imagined contexts that the patient might encounter in daily life. Gestures and other forms of nonverbal communication (accompanied by music) are part of musically assisted speech learning.

### Melodic intonation therapy (MIT)

This is a formal protocol that is similar to musically assisted speech, and has gained wide acceptance in the treatment of expressive aphasia. In this therapy, patients are guided to speak by first humming and then "intoning" target phrases to a speech-like rhythm, while tapping that rhythm with their left hand.

The word "intonation" refers to the melodic rise and fall of the voice in ordinary speech. Part of the way we convey meaning or emotion is by altering the pitch of our voice within a narrow range. In melodic intonation therapy, the person with aphasia is not singing as one might in the delivery of a Broadway aria or popular song; they are intoning—half-singing, half-speaking or chanting melodically. In so doing, they are drawing on those intact brain resources for music processing that can be rerouted to restore speech production.

The music therapist will begin with a common two-syllable word or phrase, such as "Hello," or "Let's go," using a sound pattern of *low to high* or *high to low*. The two tones or pitches will be within the patient's comfortable vocal range, and close together (technically speaking, a minor third, as from middle C to the A just below, an interval that is natural in speech) (Norton *et al.*, 2009). The intoning will approximate speech in that generally the stressed syllables will be intoned on the higher of the two pitches.

Together, the therapist and patient will practice the simple two-syllable word or phrase, while the patient taps with the left hand. Typically, the therapist's participation will fade out, as the patient continues with the exercise. As the patient improves in fluidity and expression, longer phrases are attempted using the same two tones: for example, "Let's go" becomes "Let's go/out-side." Longer constructions are possible.

A landmark study by Gottfried Schlaug, MD, PhD (2007), showed that after ten months of intensive melodic intonation therapy, the majority of patients recovered speech—and those who did showed increases in the size of the right hemisphere. This suggests that complementary or parallel networks were recruited in the right hemisphere, which supports music processing, to compensate for lost language function.

## "This little light of mine:" The story of Gabby Giffords

As many of us remember, Congresswoman Gabrielle ("Gabby") Giffords of Arizona was shot, at close range, in a mass shooting that took place at a constituent event more than ten years ago (in January, 2011). The bullet passed through the left side of Giffords' brain, leaving her partly paralyzed on the right side of her body, and unable to speak.

Giffords sustained a traumatic brain injury (TBI), with damage to Broca's area. She was diagnosed with expressive aphasia, which meant that though she could not speak, she could comprehend the speech of others. She was a prime candidate for music therapy. In the months following her injury, she began to work with a music therapist at TIRR Memorial Hermann, in Houston, Texas, in the top-tier brain injury rehabilitation program. Giffords received melodic intonation therapy. She also sang familiar songs with the music therapist, who prompted her to fill in the words to familiar lyrics.

In the years since this devastating injury, Giffords regained her speech. She has been able to speak to the media about her experience, and speak publicly, too, as a national advocate for gun control and the prevention of gun violence. She still needs to practice what she wants to say, but her speech continues to improve.

ABC News was among the media outlets that brought her story to the larger public. The media headline was "Gabby Giffords: Finding words through song," and the subheading was "How melody and rhythm can rewire the damaged brain." That, in essence, was the story.

In an ABC video, Giffords is shown, early in her therapy, unable to say the word "light." We feel her struggle, feel her tears. And then, we see her singing "This little light of mine, I'm gonna let it shine." And it does.

Watch Gabby Giffords as she finds her voice through music therapy at www.imnf.org/mhp-book-resources.

### Rhythmic cueing

Both musically assisted speech and melodic intonation therapy incorporate rhythm cueing in important ways. Therapists and patients not only intone and sing together: they also tap out songs and phrases. This is not surprising.

Speech has rhythm, and part of what needs to be restored, in people with expressive aphasia, is speech rhythm. In therapy, the patient works hard to overcome pauses, false starts, and a halting manner. Music therapists who work with aphasia patients will often clap or tap the desired speech rhythm on a drum or other surface positioned nearby, as a way of giving regular cues to a phrase that is being practiced. (If the patient doesn't understand this practice, the music therapist may begin by tapping on the patient's wrist.) Patients themselves may clap or tap on the drum the speech rhythm to the phrase that is practiced. (Patients are always advised to tap with the left hand, which engages the undamaged right hemisphere. Patients who don't have right-hand paralysis as a result of the stroke may tap with both hands, on their knees; and this too is effective.)

For rhythmic exercises, the music therapist may use song-lyric phrases, everyday conversational phrases, or phrases that are related to the immediate situation. Rhythmic cues may include slow steady beats that are gauged to the patient's speech tempo, and rhythms that are keyed to song lyrics or spoken phrases. To observe how rhythmic cueing is used in music therapy for expressive aphasia, visit www.imnf.org/mhp-book-resources.

### Breathing and oral motor exercises

Speech involves movement, and so speech rehabilitation includes exercises to improve posture, breathing and breath support, and "oral motor control," meaning control of mouth, tongue, and facial movements. For example, facial and mouth movements are demonstrated by the music therapist (often in an exaggerated way), and mirrored by the patient as they sing familiar songs. Breathing exercises help patients warm up before vocalizing, and improve their articulation (the clarity of what they want to say). Music therapists often partner with speech-language pathologists in providing breathing and movement exercises.

### Music therapy groups for people with expressive aphasia

The Institute for Music and Neurologic Function at Wartburg, and a few other progressive senior care programs, offer music therapy groups for people with expressive aphasia. The goal is to enhance speech and communication (through every means) among stroke and TBI survivors with language losses. The groups, as in individual therapy, begin with the singing of familiar songs.

A music therapist who was instrumental in developing IMNF aphasia groups described the singing that takes place in the group as a collective form of expression—deeply therapeutic for stroke patients who have suddenly found themselves unable to communicate with others in their environment.

> The patients were now looking at one another, displaying emotional facial expressions, looking at me [the therapist], and responding to shared musical events related to tempo and rhythm, lyrics and melody. We started and ended together and for the most part sang in synchrony. (Ramsey, 2002)

Music therapy groups for people with aphasia are often conceived as "support groups" for patients and their family members in the community who are dealing with post-stroke or TBI aphasia issues. And these groups often fulfill this role, first by creating a communal experience. Music helps members of the group communicate and interact with one another; and what is learned and practiced in the group can facilitate conversation with family members and friends.

Groups are generally limited to five members, and meet for 45 minutes twice a week. The music therapy includes vocal warm-up, singing of familiar songs, vocal exercises, and musically assisted phrases to facilitate simple conversations around everyday topics, such as favorite foods or sports, culminating in a communal experience.

## A music protocol for people with expressive aphasia and their care partners

The interventions used by music therapists can be adapted by family care partners, home health aides, and others, to give people with aphasia the opportunity to practice between sessions. Regular practice reinforces the therapeutic work of the session, and may accelerate recovery. And not only that: working together in music-based exercises may also increase in-sync communication between the person with aphasia and their care partner, and improve motivation and self-expression in both partners.

Here are some steps the care partners can take to provide music-based exercises for people with expressive aphasia:

- First, both partners—the care partner and the person with aphasia— must have a clear sense of the goals of the music therapy in progress, week by week (and if possible, session by session). *In other words, what skills should be practiced?* Generally, the main skills to be improved are:

  - initiation—being able to initiate speech, as evidenced by filling in words within lyrics (first the last words of each song line, then the inner words); starting a song with a cue, followed by starting a song without a cue

  - word retrieval—for example, identifying objects and colors; filling in words in practice phrases

  - speaking in short sentences (with nouns, verbs, and object, as appropriate).

- The care partner should be well informed about the music content of the session: Which songs (or phrases) are used in the session? Is there one particular song for which the goal is to sing 100 percent of the lyrics? Does the music therapist recommend introducing familiar songs that have not been used in a session?

- Set up the session as follows:

  - Sit face to face with the person who has aphasia ("the patient").

  - Ask the patient to sing with you.

  - Sing a familiar song, such as "Happy Birthday," "You Are My Sunshine," "The Alphabet Song," "Mary Had a Little Lamb," while tapping out the rhythm of the words. Tap with your right hand to mirror the patient, who is tapping with the left hand.

  - Maintain eye contact while gesturing the patient to sing and tap along with you.

  - Keep the music simple. It is best to use voice only, without instrumental accompaniment.

  - Repeat the same song several times to increase the opportunities for the person with aphasia to sing the correct words.

  - When the patient sings the song with 100 percent of the words in the lyrics, have the patient *speak* the words while tapping the rhythm.

  - You may also want to acknowledge the progress made, and provide some kind of enjoyable closure for the session.

## Other aphasias
### Wernicke's area and fluent aphasia

Many areas of the brain are known to play an important role in speech, language processing, and communication. Consequently, there are many types of aphasia, resulting from damage to different language areas and the connections between them.

We have seen that damage to Broca's area results in expressive or non-fluent aphasia—an inability to turn thoughts into spoken words. But that is only part of what may be at risk in a stroke or TBI that affects the left hemisphere. Receptive language abilities, such as the ability to understand speech as it is spoken or written, may also be affected.

About ten years after Broca identified the brain area responsible for speech production, Carl Wernicke, a German physician and psychiatrist, discovered the brain area responsible for the comprehension of speech. Wernicke had patients who were able to speak fluently, with normal rhythm and grammar, but they did not make sense. They made up or omitted words, and seemed to be unaware of the difficulties that others had in understanding them. They did not understand what others said to them. In short, they had profound difficulties in comprehending language—and not just spoken language. People with damage to Wernicke's area also had difficulties reading and writing, and sometimes making calculations as well.

In carrying out autopsies, Wernicke discovered that these patients had suffered damage to an area located, in most people, in the left hemisphere, at the back of the temporal lobe (which is involved in auditory processing, or hearing). This area came to be called "Wernicke's area," and the language disorder resulting from damage to this area is called Wernicke's aphasia, or fluent aphasia (because patients speak fluently, though they are unable to understand spoken and written language).

Because comprehension is impaired in those with fluent aphasia, the music therapy techniques used for expressive aphasia do not work well. The music therapist may encourage vocal improvisation as a means of self-expression and provide opportunities for interpersonal exchange.

## Music therapy for people with dysarthria

Dysarthria is a *motor speech problem* that may affect a person who has had a stroke, or who has a chronic disease such as multiple sclerosis or Parkinson's disease. The word "dysarthria" combines the prefix "dys," meaning "difficult," with "arthron," a Greek word meaning "joint or articulation." A person with dysarthria finds it difficult to articulate words, to pronounce them clearly, and join them together in a way that is intelligible to another person.

In dysarthria, the problem does not originate from any difficulty with language itself; people with dysarthria (unlike some people with aphasia) understand language. They are able to find and say the right words, and put them in the right order. What is missing is the *motor coordination* that is necessary to produce clear and intelligible speech. Dysarthrias (there are several kinds) are caused by damage to those areas of the brain that control the motor or movement aspects of speech, for example the muscles that move the lips and tongue, the lungs and respiratory system.

People with dysarthria often have poor breath support; when speaking they may run out of air, resulting in slurred words and poor phrasing. Words may run together; and the natural pauses between syllables and phrases may be lost or distorted. While single words are often intelligible, longer phrases or sentences present difficulties for the people with dysarthria and those with whom they would communicate. In some important way, the natural rhythm of speech is lost. In addition, certain expressive qualities of speech may be distorted. The voice may operate at one volume level (too soft or too loud)—or even at a single pitch. In a sense, the melody of speech, as well as its natural rhythm, is compromised in dysarthria. Music therapy offers a way of retrieving the sense of rhythm and melody that characterizes normal speech.

People with dysarthria are typically referred to individual speech therapy sessions, where they learn intelligibility techniques (or ways to make their speech understood by others). With practice, patients first learn to clearly say target words and phrases in brief structured exchanges such as they are likely to have with others in their environment ("How are you?" and "Thank you"). However, many patients have trouble in carrying over these techniques in actual conversations. These patients may be referred to a music therapy group, in which the focus is on restoring rhythm and the other expressive cues that make speech intelligible (Tomaino & Wilkens, 1996).

In a music therapy group, people with dysarthria learn to use musical phrases to provide a pattern for spoken phrases. Here's how it works:

- The music therapist, along with the speech-language pathologist, select a target phrase (or phrases) that can be set to a familiar melody. For example, "Hello. How are you today?" can be set to "Swing Low, Sweet Chariot." The melody matches the target phrase(s) in having the same number of syllables, the same rhythmic emphasis for these syllables, and the same pauses between syllables or words. The melody thus reflects the natural flow of the phrase(s) as spoken.

- In this protocol, the group members start by singing or chanting the original song lyrics until the lyrics are intelligible; then the target phrase is substituted. Often, small drums are used to reinforce the rhythm. Once participants have a sense of the music pattern of the phrase, longer phrases are introduced.

- To help group members master longer, multisyllabic phrases, the phrases are first divided into rhythmic groups. The music therapist is able to accentuate rhythmic patterning and demonstrate how each phrase should be spoken. As therapy progresses, members work toward achieving intelligibility in spontaneous speech. And in the long run, patients use the techniques that they have learned, even in the absence of music.

Group music therapy for people with dysarthria has been shown to support participants' sense of rhythm and melody in a way that makes it possible for them to improve articulation, phrasing, breath control, and overall intelligibility of speech. As with other speech impairments, the goal is to help patients recover, through music, essential speech functions that are closely related to our lifelong experience of music.

# Music in the Time of Covid:
# Challenges and Opportunities

The Covid-19 pandemic revealed much about the importance of social engagement for health and well-being. And it exposed the many challenges facing healthcare delivery systems. How much does social interaction affect our mental health? How do people access health-related services? And what happens when social interaction is restricted, when social supports go missing, and people are unable to access health-related services through the usual channels?

In early 2020, once Covid-19 lockdowns were in place, the challenges in accessing care became strikingly obvious. In skilled nursing and assisted living facilities all residents were confined to their rooms. There were no group programs. Only basic needs were being provided for. Everywhere, here and around the world, people were confined to their homes. The impact of isolation and fear became omnipresent.

But then something remarkable happened. People started singing from balconies, front porches, and fire-escapes, sharing music with their neighbors. They were using music as a way to stay connected and deal with the emotional strain of isolation.

## The impact of music engagement

Research on the impact of music engagement during Covid-19 lockdowns showed an increase in use of music—both listening to and making music—as a means of coping. Several research studies, conducted during the first year of the Covid-19 pandemic, examined the variety of ways that people used music. These studies showed the importance of real-time musical responses to a social crisis, as well as individual adaptations in music-related behaviors to meet social and emotional needs.

One study revealed that people who experienced an increase in negative emotions during lockdown listened to music to relieve feelings of depression, stress, and fear. Those with a more positive state of mind turned to music as a replacement for social interaction (Fink *et al.*, 2021).

The internet and technology made connections possible in ways not utilized before. We found that there are both benefits and challenges in accessing programs and music via the internet. Issues around bandwidth, connectivity, equipment, and access to wifi are important in that they can help or hinder someone's ability to benefit from online programs. Nevertheless, **virtual programs provided access to music for many people who previously had not been able to participate in live programs, either due to limited programs in their area or transportation and mobility issues**. Put simply, many people who were unable to attend in-person sessions were able to access music therapy on Zoom or other online platforms. Online programs increased participation and satisfaction in ways we could not have previously imagined.

The variety of ways people engaged in music included the following:

- Listening to music

- Dancing

- Singing

- Participating in a chorus

- Playing an instrument

- Sharing music videos and stories

- Listening to or sharing pre-recorded programs

- Attending Facebook Live programs

- Attending music-based Zoom activities.

People were also able to access therapeutic music programming, including:

- Music therapy sessions online (or on Zoom)

- Music therapy groups online (or on Zoom) for special populations (e.g. people with PTSD, aphasia, Parkinson's disease, dementia)

- Music-based groups for mental health and wellness online (or on Zoom).

The impact of virtual programs was highlighted in a major population survey that found that music helped people relax and "escape," improved mood, boosted confidence and coping ability, reduced the sense of isolation, and improved connectivity with others (Cabedo-Mas *et al.*, 2021).

## Adaptations for assisted living and skilled nursing facilities

During the first 18 months or so of the Covid-19 pandemic, residents of assisted living and nursing home facilities were isolated in their own rooms. No community programs were permitted. Later, music programs became possible in courtyards or hallways, with residents keeping their distance by staying at the door of their rooms.

Virtual programs became possible as we provided Facebook Live programs or Zoom sessions that could be viewed on a large smart TV. In cases where residents needed to be isolated, a staff member brought a digital tablet to each individual and turned on the Facebook Live program, if the resident couldn't access it on their own. Though this was time consuming for the staff member, it was one of the only ways to provide more directed programs to individual residents.

Facilities that had internal TV stations were able to stream live programs. At Wartburg, which was fortunate to have such a setup, musicians regularly performed in the chapel, and the performance was broadcasted to the various residences on campus. The only staff requirement was for a CNA or therapeutic recreation specialist to turn on the resident's in-room TV to the in-house station.

In this way, it was possible to provide, to many isolated residents, music that gave pleasure, solace, and strength, while creating a shared music experience across the community.

### Zooming ahead

Zoom and other conferencing platforms became ubiquitous among online programs; and these platforms soon enhanced the options due to increased demand. Zoom provided a platform that allowed individual music therapy sessions to continue, and Zoom sessions were shown to be very effective in supporting music therapy goals—for example, enhancing cognitive skills through reminiscence and singing. Through Zoom, people who had participated in a group program prior to Covid-19 could continue to connect to group members. Seeing one another on the screen contributed to the sense of participating in a group program even though everyone was isolated in their own homes. Seeing the faces of group friends helped maintain a sense of togetherness. (Note that for people with dementia, seeing too many faces on screen may be confusing, and it can be better to leave the screen on speaker view.)

By sharing a screen, the music therapist or group leader could share YouTube videos of Frank Sinatra at the Paramount or Chuck Berry at the Apollo, immediately triggering recall and memory associations for remote participants. Each shared memory can lead to another similar music selection and question prompts; for example, "Did you go to the Apollo?" "Who else did you see there?" "Did you know that Ella Fitzgerald performed there?" "Do you like her songs?" "Which one?" Each question draws the participant further into the experience and provides an opportunity for the music therapist or group leader to evaluate how best to engage that participant. Setting up the Zoom ahead of time so that "share computer audio" is selected is important. Also important is turning off advertisements, as these are not only disruptive to the flow of the program but may be inappropriate at times.

During the Covid-19 pandemic, creative arts organizations found ways to provide concerts online, including opportunities to interact with musicians in Q&As after the performance. Other organizations created pre-recorded programming especially for seniors, such as music and exercise, music meditation, and music for relaxation.

## TAKEAWAYS

The biggest TAKEAWAY from the Covid-19 pandemic was how many people could be reached through online programs, and how these online connections could serve as a lifeline to maintain health and combat isolation, depression, and mental decline. As challenging as social isolation was during Covid-19, it revealed an enormous need that could be met through technology. Social isolation has always been an issue with older adults, and has actually been identified as a huge health risk. Even with in-person programs now possible there will still be people who cannot attend for a variety of reasons. With technology and virtual programs we can now come to them and remove barriers (such as transportation or mobility issues) that would otherwise prevent them from participating. Virtual programs will continue to expand and new online platforms will be developed that will enable greater access to music engagement.

A TAKEAWAY for music therapists was that music therapy, which was not widely available to older people, and music therapy-informed activities, which had been available as part of a patchwork of recreational activities, if at all, might now be offered online to a much larger population—conceivably to anyone with an internet connection.

# Technology and Virtual Programming: Expanding Access to Music Therapy and Music Programming

This section is supported by an *Online Technology Resource Guide* at www. imnf.org/mhp-book-resources.

More than 25 years ago, the IMNF was established to advance the best practices in music therapy through research, education, and training. Music Has Power® became our message and our "brand." Our mission was, and is, to develop and deliver effective treatments to awaken, stimulate, and heal through the extraordinary powers of music.

Today, music has more power than ever, because you have power too. With access to wifi and internet services, almost anyone can access music in every genre and time period, including live videos of artists performing their hit songs. Music-based technologies are enabling people without any music training to make music and interact musically with others—even to compose their own music.

Seniors are among those who benefit. A review of research suggests that older people, even those with complex needs, are capable of, and interested in, using music technologies to access and create personally meaningful music (Creech, 2019). Technology can help older adults access their favorite music—for reminiscence, to support singing, to support music perception and appreciation, to engage in collaborative music-making, and to facilitate music and movement activities.

Caregivers play an important role in helping patients and loved ones access music and the therapeutic power of music. **In senior care, music technology users include caregivers and patients at all levels of physical, emotional, and neurologic function. Technology has accelerated the** delivery of music, with all its therapeutic potential, to seniors in nursing homes and other residential settings, and to seniors cared for at home, or living independently in the community.

## Music technology is about now—and the future

In this section of the book, we will offer an overview of the technologies used to introduce therapeutic music into senior healthcare (as well as healthcare settings generally). For practical reasons, we will focus on mainstream technology—that is, the kinds of devices and apps that are currently available, and in many cases free to use.

But technology is constantly being upgraded, and reinvented. Many of the devices mentioned will be around for a while, but the apps and delivery services may change. The *Online Technology Resource Guide*, available at www.imnf.org/mhp-book-resources, will provide the most up-to-date information on devices and apps related to caregiving and senior health and wellness. This resource will help you choose among available options, to bring meaningful music experiences to yourself and those in your care.

## A music therapy perspective on music technology

Music technology has transformed everything. It has brought the joy of music, and the healing power of music, to everyone with an internet connection (which is a large part of the world). But...

Music technology is not in itself therapeutic: to achieve therapeutic goals, technology must be designed to be easily used by the targeted user *with therapeutic intent*. **The music technology user—whether a music therapist or caregiver, a patient or well senior—must receive guidance, and, ideally, training, both in the use of the technology, and in music therapy best practices.** Therapeutic intent shapes the use we make of technological devices, and what we are able to achieve.

For example, we have referred to the ways in which technology can deliver a familiar song that unlocks memories, moods, and feelings of a person with dementia. If you are a caregiver, streaming apps will help you select music for your patient, based on the filters you apply (which are themselves based on music therapy research). But these tools do not guarantee success. The music therapist, caregiver, or family care partner must provide *the right music for the person, at the right time*. Training in music therapy best practices helps caregivers select music that supports caregiving and meets the needs of patients, in the moment. Technology alone cannot do this.

**For music interventions to be effective, a therapeutic relationship must**

be established between caregivers and patients, if only for the moment. The shared interaction around music in real time is what is most likely to be therapeutic—*however* that experience is delivered.

In 2010, the public was transfixed by the YouTube video of Henry, a person with dementia who was awakened by hearing his favorite music on an iPod (see Module 5). Henry's awakening went viral, as evidence of the power of music; what was less noted was that Henry was supported by caregivers who knew his life history and interacted with him as he listened to his favorite music. For patients like Henry, a familiar song, pulled from a streaming service or an iPod playlist, will work best if caregivers are present—to engage with the patient and their family through the music, to encourage communication of feelings and memories, or simply to be there in the moment.

The same holds true for the use of other music technologies that have the potential to deliver a therapeutic experience. A smart TV, tuned to potentially therapeutic programming—say, songs from the 1950s, or popular showtunes—will not have the intended effect if the program is simply turned on for a group of patients in a day room while caregivers attend to tasks elsewhere. The presence of one CNA or volunteer to help deliver the program—to call out residents by name and urge them to clap or sing along—will help deliver the experience. The power of music, as therapy, almost always depends on a therapeutic relationship, if only in the moment.

Training in music therapy best practices helps build therapeutic relationships that are realized through technology support.

## Expanding access: A core value

Throughout this book, the role of technology has been integrated into music therapy best practice. Here we explore the role of technology in *expanding access* to music therapy, and to music programming that has been shown to benefit seniors in residential care, and in the community.

Expanding access to music therapy is a core value of the IMNF, and of the field of music therapy in general. We believe that:

- everyone can benefit from music; and those with neurologic and neurocognitive challenges should have access to music therapy

- technology accelerates the delivery of therapeutic aspects of music to benefit those who have limited access to music therapy

- collaboration with technology companies, technology researchers, and entrepreneurs advances our mission.

## Music-making: "We are all musicians"

Music therapy, as a treatment modality, seeks to be inclusive and accessible to people at all levels of function. From the beginning, technological innovation has helped us realize this mission.

Music therapists were among the first to adapt conventional musical instruments for people with physical impairments—adding grips to handheld instruments, refitting keyboards—improvising wherever possible. In time, technology provided specialized electronic instruments that were designed to reach a diverse population of patients with special needs. Among these early instruments were electronic triggers (called piezo triggers). Placed on a drum surface, the triggers convert stimuli into a computer language that is sent to a converter to produce sound. The triggers are easily activated by patients with limited strength and fine motor skills. Soundbeam, another early example, is a touch-free device that uses ultrasonic sensors to allow patients with little or no arm movement to produce musical sounds—and music—with a nod of the head or a small wave of the hand.

As early as the mid-90s, specialized electronic instruments were used by IMNF music therapists in the treatment of patients affected by stroke, traumatic brain injury (TBI), amputations, and other physical and sensory impairments. Technological advances continued to expand access to music therapy, where music therapy was offered.

*Fast forward*, and today a dazzling array of electronic devices, music-based apps, and virtual instruments is available—not just for people with special needs, but for *anyone who might want to make music*. Collaborations between music therapists, technology companies, and the music products industry have made this happen.

Everyone is empowered: because, for the most part, digital music devices require minimal dexterity, skill, or strength. The music-maker can simply tap on a touch screen to play a few notes. On a guitar app, for example, playing chords in every key is as simple as pressing the chord button; to strum a chord, the music-maker can tap on the desired string or use a sweeping motion, as with a real guitar. In short, **music technology available today provides the immediate capability to make music that can take years to acquire on conventional (acoustic) instruments** (Magee, 2013). We should note that music-making includes singing. Technology platforms also offer enjoyable "failure free" singing, for people with dementia and other challenges. Available apps can help tune your voice to the correct notes, and provide accompaniment.

Apps and software provide a wealth of musical ideas and options that can often be mastered on a "short learning curve." Wendy Magee, PhD, BMus, who has studied music technology in healthcare settings, notes that "for people dealing with fatigue, cognitive slowing due to medication, anxiety or other emotional difficulties, or reduced physical dexterity, music technologies provide immediate success and access to becoming 'a musician'" (2013, p.364).

The short learning curve makes music technology accessible to caregivers as well.

## "Personalized music"—for people with dementia, for everyone

In this book, we have explored the therapeutic value of familiar songs in dementia care, and in individual and group therapy for people with dementia, speech disorders, and mental health and wellness issues.

Forty years ago, familiar songs were used, to great effect, by the very few music therapists who worked in senior care settings, to treat a very few patients. The therapist identified songs with personal meaning to the person with dementia, and proceeded to sing the songs, live, with guitar or piano accompaniment. We observed that the music could have an "almost magical" effect on people with dementia, by eliciting memories and associations, and restoring the moods, memories, and feelings of their former selves.

We saw that the moment when the magic happens was very special: but that it did not extend beyond the session. ("You are the music, while the music lasts," says the poet T.S. Eliot). But after that? What was needed was for these moments to happen on a more regular basis, as part of everyday life. Being on full-time staff, I was able to work every day with people with memory problems and saw how consistent engagement in music-based activities improved their short-term memory as well as social engagement. But my situation was unique, as most skilled nursing facilities don't have full-time music therapists on staff. The consistent engagement was and is necessary for any carry-over benefits.

*Fast forward*, and with the arrival of the MP3 and later the Apple iPods, it became easy to store familiar songs in portable media players, making therapeutic music immediately accessible to people everywhere, including people in long-term care settings. With this new technology, **personalized playlists could be delivered, on a daily basis, by caregivers in memory care and long-term care settings. A patient's favorite music could be integrated with everyday care, to elicit memories, create a positive mood, and reduce anxiety and difficult behaviors.** CNAs and other caregivers could be trained to deliver music for bath time and bedtime, music to encourage participation in dressing and grooming cooperation with wound care, and much more. Experience and research showed that using playlists and personalized music in dementia care resulted in benefits to both patients and caregiving staff.

Today, the use of personalized playlists in dementia care is well established in the US and other nations with a robust music therapy practice (including the UK, Canada, Australia, and Norway).

In the US, the nonprofit organization Music & Memory has led the way in introducing personalized playlists or iPod programs for dementia patients. Founded in 2010, Music & Memory has seeded programs in 5800 healthcare sites to date; and that number does not account for total US programming. In a very few years we have seen a tremendous expansion in the access to personalized music for people with dementia—thanks, in part, to MP3c, iPods, tablets, and iPhones.

Music therapy best practices in the use of personalized playlists and other forms of personal music in dementia care are described in Modules 5 and 6. Other uses of personalized playlists appear throughout the book. We suggest—we expect—that CNAs and other caregivers will put together their own playlists, to support personal wellness goals. Because personalized playlists have become part of our broader music culture, people of all ages, at all levels of function, rely on their favorite music, accessible on portable digital devices and online platforms, to manage their moods and meet wellness needs.

## Expanded access through telemedicine and virtual programs

In response to a nationwide shortage of music therapists, the IMNF began, some years ago, to treat patients remotely, on telemedicine platforms such as Skype, Zoom, and Facebook. During the Covid-19 pandemic, online therapy of every kind became the only option for many of those needing service—and technology stepped up to meet the demand. Not surprisingly, the demand was for therapy that helped people cope with isolation, depression, and other challenges posed by the pandemic.

Zoom and similar platforms hosted individual music therapy sessions, as well as the therapeutic group work that is more often undertaken in healthcare settings. At the IMNF, for example, we continued to offer individual sessions for people with speech disorders and memory issues, remotely, and beyond our own community. We also offered group sessions on the Zoom platform—a "hybrid" in-person and virtual model—for veterans with PTSD, patients with Parkinson's disease and their care partners, and patients with expressive aphasia and their care partners. In long-term care, where patients were isolated in their rooms, Zoom sessions helped residents connect to group members and maintain cognitive skills through reminiscence and singing.

The Covid-19 pandemic shined a bright light on the role of technology in delivering music interventions; but the need and demand for supportive technology had been there all along. Given the shortage of music therapists, there has always been a significant population with little access to music therapy—and a healthcare workforce with limited access to the therapeutic benefits that music can provide. Zoom and other virtual programs that became ubiquitous during the pandemic expanded access in ways we could easily see, but they were part of a much larger picture.

## Expanded options for in-person music interventions in care settings

Technology has also helped increase access to in-person music-based groups for seniors in residential care and adult day programs. The driving force here, as generally, has been technology that allows recreation therapists, CNAs, and others to access music resources with therapeutic intent.

Smart TVs, installed in the day rooms of long-term care facilities, allow easy access to internet searches, YouTube, and streaming services. With training in music therapy best practices, staff can use these resources in group programs, such as singalongs or music reminiscence programs. Karaoke and music videos are also easily accessible. For the recreation therapist or CNA, an added benefit is that smart TVs allow screen-sharing from a tablet or phone directly to the smart TV monitor, enabling the group leader to program activity content in advance of a session.

Streaming services such as Spotify, Apple Music, and Sound Cloud also support recreation therapists and CNAs in leading group programs. These streaming services (and the internet generally) make it easy for a group leader to access songs requested on the spot. No longer is it necessary for the leader to be able to play music of all genres, live, as music therapists are trained to do. Although something is lost with the widespread use of pre-recorded music (which cannot be altered or improvised to meet immediate needs), much is gained by making music, performed to high musical standards, available on demand to groups that are led by non-musicians.

## Are we all music composers, too?

Music therapists are trained to partner with patients in composing music that achieves therapeutic goals. For example, a music therapist may support a patient in composing music that expresses feelings the patient cannot express in words, which then become a focus of therapy. Music apps allow music composition to be offered primarily as a creative activity—and the results may be therapeutic or just plain fun. Recreation therapists and CNAs with music background or interests can use apps such as Garageband and BandLab to help patients create music passages and compositions, in support of wellness goals (such as increasing self-esteem and creativity); mental health goals (overcoming social isolation and depression symptoms); and rehabilitation goals. These apps make it easy to select a music style, such as swing, rock, pop, ballad, Latin. The rhythmic pattern and potential harmonies are generated by the app and can be used as background to the songwriting activity. Musician volunteers are often excellent partners in music composition, with or without apps.

Recording and sharing one's composition may be part of the creative or therapeutic process. A few pioneering music therapy programs, the IMNF among them, have set up "recording studios" for patients in rehabilitation and long-term care. Emerging technology makes recording and production facilities more feasible for healthcare facilities. In the past, special recording, mixing, and editing equipment was needed. Today this can be done with a laptop or tablet, with the proper software or app.

## The new music therapy-informed workforce

By making music and music-making accessible to everyone, technology has expanded the healthcare workforce that can be trained to deliver music interventions in line with music therapy best practices.

The magic formula is *Technology + Training = Expanded access.*

Although music technologies—the latest devices—are designed to be used with ease by the largest possible audience, training is required to use these devices with therapeutic intent. Training is most successful when it is developed by music therapists in collaboration with other healthcare professionals, administrators, and educators.

For example, it's a fairly simple matter to collect favorite songs on a personalized playlist. Yet the 5800 healthcare sites that use Music & Memory iPod programs provide trainings (with certification) to ensure that staff are empowered to use the playlist in line with music therapy best practices. Only about 100 of the healthcare organizations certified by Music & Memory have music therapists on staff. In other words, technology plus training has greatly increased access to therapeutic music, for hundreds of thousands of people with dementia who have never seen a music therapist.[1]

---

[1]  Disclosure: both the author and the President/CEO of Wartburg serve on the Board of Directors for Music & Memory.

## Access to training
### Formal training programs
Training in the use of music technology for therapeutic purposes can be acquired through formal training programs and certifications, through in-service workshops conducted by music therapists, and through guide-books on music therapy best practices, such as this. In most cases, training will incorporate videos that show music interventions delivered by music therapists or trained caregiving staff.

Long-term care facilities that have well-developed music therapy pro-grams may publish and distribute their own training materials to both staff and family care partners; typically, these trainings focus on using music and music technology in the everyday care of people with Alzheimer's and other forms of dementia. But there are other possibilities: for example, trainings might focus on the everyday care of people who have depression symptoms, or people who are inactive, unresponsive to care, or resistant to rehabilitation.

Specialized training guides and videos are available for community-based interventions, such as therapeutic drum circles, ballroom dancing, and cho-ruses for people with dementia and their care partners.

### Online training experiences
Online courses and other computer-based learning experiences have tended to focus on dementia care, targeting family care partners as well as professional caregivers. Accessed on computers and other digital devices, these online courses show caregivers how to deliver music interventions, often using widely accessible technology (iPhones, tablets, and other easy-to-use devices, music apps, apps for music streaming, voice assistants, and more). **Especially in dementia care, mainstream technology has expanded the workforce that can deliver music interventions.** It is up to music therapists and caregivers to step up to the task: training materials must recognize that technology is only a tool, and that care, or therapy, involves an understanding of the whole person, the nature and course of dementia, and music therapy best practices.

Nonprofit organizations, including senior-serving and disease-specific organizations, often provide web-based guidance and resources on the use of therapeutic music for their communities. Such organizations include, for example, the Alzheimer's Foundation of America, which provides caregiver workshops, and Music Mends Minds, which advocates for opportunities for musicians and singers with memory challenges to continue to rehearse and perform. Internet searches will discover many resources, from many sources. Insofar as these sources are informed by music therapists and music therapy best practices, they raise awareness and help expand access to therapeutic music.

## Training apps for family care partners and professional caregivers

Music therapy researchers and their project teams are developing and testing mobile apps that help caregivers use music to improve everyday care for people with dementia. The apps are designed to be used by family care partners, on their own. In the best cases, navigating the program is simple; step-by-step guidance, and sometimes feedback, is part of the program. One cutting-edge app uses integrated sensors to "learn" the typical behavioral patterns of the person with dementia, and guides the caregiver in matching the music to the person's needs in the moment. Another works on face and voice tone recognition to determine the emotional state of the person with dementia, and to direct caregiver responses accordingly. The cutting edge moves as we step forward, so we can expect that technology will continue to deliver new products to support caregivers in using music in dementia care, because the need—the market—is very large, and growing.

## Collaborations with technology companies and the music industry

Training may be provided directly by technology companies that work closely with music therapists in monitoring and improving product use. For example, a representative of the company that designed the music-enhanced treadmill used in gait training (see "Digital music technology: The musically enhanced treadmill" in Module 7) regularly visited the IMNF rehabilitation gym to work with music therapists, physical therapists, and occupational therapists. Collaboration involved problem-solving, learning, and building "bridges of understanding" among staff and patients who interacted with the technology (Wilcox, D., occupational therapist, personal communication, May 3, 2022). Technology companies that design music technology for specific patient populations often collaborate with music therapists and neuroscience researchers to build their products; and guidance for the effective use of these products is built into marketing efforts, which may reach a wide audience.

Some technology and music industry companies have gone into the training business themselves. Though this seems a recent trend, it should not surprise us. Remo, Inc., a leading manufacturer of drums and drumheads, has developed numerous training products focused on drum circles and rhythm activities, in collaboration with music therapists, musicians, and communities. Today Remo, Inc. offers—you guessed it—free weekly online live drum circle experiences from your home, on Zoom.

## Partnering with patients and care partners to increase the impact of music therapy

For health organizations that provide music therapy services, technology helps augment those services. **Patients and care partners can be trained to use music therapeutically between sessions—thus increasing the impact of music therapy.**

For example, people with Parkinson's disease typically receive therapy in the rehabilitation gym. For gait training, the music therapist may prescribe music with a specific tempo, observing and fine-tuning the rhythm and pace during the session. Once a safe, optimal walking tempo is established, the music therapist will ask the patient for the types of music or songs that they enjoy. The music therapist will select from the patient's preferred songs those that fit that tempo and create a walking track that they can use at home. With access to streaming services that allow for filters on the tempo or beats per minute (BPM) and musical style, people with Parkinson's and their care partners can search for additional music selections that will be therapeutic, and they can practice at home, thus building on their in-person session with a music therapist (or physical therapist). Similarly, people treated for expressive aphasia can use an app that is programmed to run them through therapeutic exercises, in line with music therapy best practices. Online coaching can also help augment in-person music therapy between sessions.

## What's next?

Artificial intelligence applications are being developed to deliver music in healthcare settings (Foster *et al.*, 2021). Start-ups and research projects in the US, Canada, Australia, and elsewhere send news of what we might expect. "A music therapist and human-computer interaction expert help carers (care-givers) use music to calm people with dementia," announced the Australian Government in 2022, referencing the eHealth project of Felicity Baker, PhD, M.Mus, RMT, at the University of Melbourne. The project team will design the algorithm that chooses what music to play for the person with dementia, based on the person's level of agitation in real time. It is anticipated that the team will use wearable sensors to detect changes in biomarkers and behaviors in the person with dementia. The computer will automatically select and match personalized music to the agitation (or other behavior), detect the person's response, and adjust as needed. We are also likely to see artificial intelligence applications that focus on caregiver training.

Virtual reality, too, will provide new options for delivering music in healthcare contexts. For example, a US start-up called ngram promises to develop immersive experiences based on well-validated therapeutic approaches, including music therapy. These immersive experiences will be available on any phone or tablet. Projects in the works target older adults, people with dementia, caregivers, and families.

## Stay connected

For up-to-date information and additional resources, visit www.imnf.org/mhp-book-resources.

# Resources for Reference and Self-Study

## Music and the brain

*Musicophilia: Tales of Music and the Brain*, revised and expanded edition paperback, by Oliver Sacks (Vintage, 2008)

*This is your Brain on Music: The Science of a Human Obsession*, paperback, illustrated, by Daniel J. Levitin (Plume/Penguin, reprint edition, 2007)

*The World in Six Songs: How the Musical Brain Created Human Nature*, paperback, by Daniel J. Levitin (Dutton/Penguin, 2016)

*Of Sound Mind: How Our Brain Constructs a Meaningful Sonic World*, hardcover, by Nina Kraus (The MIT Press, 2021)

*Your Brain on Art: How the Arts Transform Us*, by Susan Magsamen and Ivy Ross (Random House, 2023)

## Music programs/activities with older adults

*Therapeutic Uses of Music with Older Adults* by Alicia Ann Clair, Jenny Memmott (American Music Therapy Association, second edition, 2008)

*Connecting through Music with People with Dementia: A Guide for Caregivers* by Robin Rio (Jessica Kingsley Publishers, 2009)

*Musically Engaged Seniors: 40 Session Plans and Resources for a Vibrant Music Therapy Program*, paperback, by Meredith Faith Hamons MT-BC (Whelk & Waters Publishing, 2013)

*Listen, Sing, Dance, Play: Bring Musical Moments into the Rhythms of Caregiving* by Rachelle Morgan (Ivie Sanders Publishing, 2022)

*Group Rhythm and Drumming with Older Adults: Music Therapy Techniques and Multimedia Training Guide*, paperback, by Barbara Reuer, Barbara Crowe, Barry Bernstein & Barbara Else (editors), Tawna Grasty. Grass T Design (illustrator) (American Music Therapy, 2007)

*Music, Memory, and Meaning: How to Effectively Use Music to Connect with Aging Loved Ones* by Meredith Hamons, Tara Jenkins & Cathy Befi-Hensel (Whelk & Waters Publishing, 2017)

## Music therapy

*The New Music Therapist's Handbook* by Suzanne B. Hanser (Berklee Press, third edition, 2018)

*Music Therapy: An Introduction to the Profession* by Andrew J. Knight, A. Blythe LaGasse, Alicia Ann Clair (American Music Therapy Association, 2018)

*Music Therapy in Dementia Care (Arts Therapies)*, David Aldridge (editor) (Jessica Kingsley Publishers, 2008)

*Musical Assessment of Gerontologic Needs and Treatment—The MAGNET Survey* by Roberta S. Adler (Jessica Kingsley Publishers, 2022)

*Receptive Methods in Music Therapy*, paperback, by Denise Grocke & Tony Wigram (Jessica Kingsley Publishers, illustrated edition, 2006)

*Handbook of Neurologic Music Therapy* by Michael H. Thaut & Volker Hoemberg (editors) (Oxford University Press, reprint edition, 2014)

# Acknowledgments

We are grateful to the Scott Amrhein Memorial Fund, for inspiring us with their support and helping to make this project possible. This memorial fund was established during the spring of 2020 as a way to remember and honor Scott Amrhein, founder and president of the Continuing Care Leadership of the Greater New York Hospital Association, and a lifelong drummer. We are honored to share a tribute to Scott from his family, as we continue our work, in his spirit, and with generous support.

Serving the elderly and creating music were both passions of Scott's throughout his life. In his professional work, Scott exemplified great commitment to the elderly and disabled through his leadership roles with nonprofit, long-term care providers in the New York City area. He most recently served as founder and president of the Continuing Care Leadership Coalition, an affiliate of the Greater New York Hospital Association. Scott also served as vice president of long-term care at the Greater New York Hospital Association and as a legislative assistant in health policy for the United States Senator Alfonse D'Amato.

Scott cared passionately about the needs of the elderly and disabled in our society. His work was not just a job for him, it was a true mission to help others. Scott was also passionate about music and recognized the importance of music therapy programs in long-term care settings and in individual homes. He believed music could provide comfort to people, facilitate memory care, and increase social connection with others.

As a lifetime drummer, Scott knew the connection between our brain function and music. He also knew the importance of music during periods of recovery from illnesses and surgeries. Creating ways to make music therapy more accessible, both in facilities and in individual homes, was important to Scott. He knew that our healthcare workers and caregivers were often on the frontlines of making a difference in the lives of the elderly and disabled.

It is the hope of Scott's family that this book will be a way to reach out to more people and to add joy and meaning in the lives of those who are being cared for and their caregivers. Blessings and deep appreciation are expressed for the sacred work that is done. May you enjoy the gift of music that comes from the heart.

The family of Scott Amrhein

There are so many people who helped make this book possible. I am especially grateful to Dr. David Gentner, a  champion of IMNF and its mission, whose faith in me provided the motivation to pull together all the resources I and IMNF staff have created over the years and synthesize it into this useable guide.  To Joan Brown who has been a supporter of music therapy for decades through her work with the Florence Tyson Fund for Creative Arts Therapies and a friend, grant writer and writer/editor for more than 30 years with IMNF. Without her writing and editing help this book would never have been completed.

I am thankful to Scott Amrhein, of blessed memory, who was an ardent supporter of music programs in senior care and for the grant, in his honor, from the Scott Amrhein memorial fund of the Greater New York Hospital Association (GNYHA)

I am truly thankful for the friendship and leadership of Edwin "Eddie" H. Stern, III whom I first met in the 1980's when I gave a presentation to the Beth Abraham Health Services board of directors about the promise of music therapy for people with dementia. He immediately saw its value and became the driving force to create the Institute for Music and Neurologic Function in 1995. When he became Chairman of IMNF in 2001, I had the opportunity to work alongside him to build the board of directors and the organization. His support, wisdom, and advocacy have been an enormous help to me over the years. To Arnold Goldstein, of blessed memory, who brought together the necessary support to make the IMNF a reality. I am grateful to the extraordinary IMNF board directors who have provided leadership and support. To the staff of Wartburg, especially Rose Cappa-Rotunno, for their time and expertise. I am thankful for the insights and resources from Justin Russo and Ann Wyatt of Music & Memory,® who have done so much to raise public awareness of the importance of our shared mission.  And we owe a special thanks to the terrific editorial team at Jessica Kingsley Publishers.

I am forever grateful to Oliver Sacks, of blessed memory, whose friendship and collaborations during our 35 years working together continue to inspire me.   To all the special individuals who have benefitted from music therapy along with their family members for allowing me to share their stories and from whom I have learned so much.   And most importantly I'm grateful for the endless support of my husband, Walter Barrett, and our children, Rebecca and Bernadetto.

# References

AARP (2010). How Lonely Are You? *AARP Magazine*, September 24, 2010. www.aarp. org/personal-growth/transitions/info-09-2010/How-Lonely-are-You.html.

Abbott, E. (2018). Song Transformation with Older Adults in a Skilled Nursing Facility. In A. Heiderscheit & N. Jackson, *Introduction to Music Therapy Practice* (pp.95–199). Dallas, TX: Barcelona Publishers.

Alzheimer's Association (n.d.). www.alz.org.

American Psychiatric Association (n.d.). What is Depression? www.psychiatry.org/ patients-families/depression/what-is-depression, accessed on February 26, 2023.

American Psychiatric Association (2022). *Diagnostic and Statistical Manual of Mental Disorders* (fifth edition, text rev.). https://doi.org/10.1176/appi. books.9780890425787.

Blood, A.J. & Zatorre, R.J. (2001). Intensely pleasurable responses to music correlate with activity in brain regions implicated in reward and emotion. *Proceedings of the National Academy of Sciences*, 98(20), 11818–11823. https://doi.org/10.1073/ pnas.191355898.

Bowell, S. & Bamford, S. (2018). "What would life be: Without a song or a dance, what are we?" A Report from the Commission on Dementia and Music. London: International Longevity Centre.

Brancatisano, O., Barid, A.B. & Thompson, W.F. (2020). Why is music therapeutic for neurological disorders? The Therapeutic Music Capacities Module. *Neuroscience and Biobehavioral Reviews*, 112, May 2020, 600–615. https://doi.org/10.1016/j. neubiorev.2020.02.008.

Bruscia, K.E., Hesser, B. & Boxill, E.H. (1981). Essential competencies for the practice of music therapy. *Music Therapy*, 1(1), 43–49. https://doi.org/10.1093/mt/1.1.43.

Cabedo-Mas, A., Arriaga-Sanz, C. & Moliner-Miravet, L. (2021). Uses and perceptions of music in times of COVID-19: A Spanish population survey. *Frontiers in Psychology*, 11. https://doi.org/10.3389/fpsyg.2020.606180.

CaringKind (2022). *Finding Comfort: Living with Advanced Dementia in Residential Care: A Consumer Guide*. New York, NY: CaringKind.

Centers for Disease Control and Prevention (n.d.). Stroke Facts. www.cdc.gov/stroke/ facts.htm, accessed on February 26, 2023.

Centers for Disease Control and Prevention (2014). QuickStats: *Percentage of Users of Long-Term Care Services with a Diagnosis of Depression, by Provider Type: National Study of Long-Term Care Providers, United States, 2011 and 2012*. CDC. www.cdc. gov/mmwr/preview/mmwrhtml/mm6304a7.htm, accessed on February 24, 2023.

Clair, A.A. (1996). *Therapeutic Uses of Music with Older Adults*. Baltimore, MD: Health Professions Press.

Clemons, C.N. (2021). "How Do We Respond to That Level of Need?" Supporting the Mental Health of Skilled Nursing Facility Residents in San Francisco. Long Term Care Coordinating Council, University of California, Berkeley. www.sfhsa.org/sites/default/files/Report_SNF_%2BLetter_6.24.21.pdf.

Creech, A. (2019). Using music technology creatively to enrich later-life: A literature review. *Frontiers in Psychology*, 10, 117. doi: 10.3389/fpsyg.2019.00117.

Faculty of Public Health (n.d.). Concepts of health, wellbeing and illness, and the aetiology of illness. www.healthknowledge.org.uk/public-health-textbook/medical-sociology-policy-economics/4a-concepts-health-illness/section2/activity3, accessed on October 3, 2023.

Fink, L.K., Warrenburg, L.A., Howlin, C., Randall, W.M., Hansen, N.C. & Wald-Fuhrmann, M. (2021). Viral tunes: Changes in musical behaviours and interest in coronamusic predict socio-emotional coping during COVID-19 lockdown. *Humanities and Social Sciences Communications*, 8, 180. https://doi.org/10.1057/s41599-021-00858-y.

Foster, B., Pearson, S., Berends, A. & Mackinnon, C. (2021). The expanding scope, inclusivity, and integration of music in healthcare: Recent developments, research illustration, and future direction. *Healthcare*, 9, 99. https://doi.org/10.3390/healthcare9010099.

Garrido, S., Dunne, L., Chang, E., Perz, J., Stevens, C.J. & Haertsch, M. (2017). The use of music playlists for people with dementia: A critical synthesis. *Journal of Alzheimer's Disease*, 60(3), 1129–1142. doi: 10.3233/JAD-170612.

Gentner, D.J. (2017). *Music and Dementia: A Caregiver's Perspective of the Effects of Individualized Music Programming on Quality of Life for Seniors Living in Assisted Living Environments*. Education Doctoral. Paper 305.

Gupta, S. (2021). *Keep Sharp: Build a Better Brain at Any Age*. New York, NY: Simon & Schuster.

Hackney, M.E. & Earhart, G.M. (2009). Effects of dance on movement control in Parkinson's disease: A comparison of Argentine tango and American ballroom. *Journal of Rehabilitation Medicine*, 41(6), 475–481. doi: 10.2340/16501977-0362.

Hammar, L.M. *et al.* (2010). Reactions of persons with dementia to caregivers singing in morning care situations. *Open Nursing Journal*, 4, 31–41.

Hanc, J. (2021). "Doctors are prescribing ways to connect socially for those feeling isolated." *The New York Times*, May 25, 2021.

Hart, M. (1991). Statement at Forever Young: Music and Aging, Hearing before the Special Committee on Aging, United States Senate, 102nd Congress, First Session; Washington, DC, August 1, 1991.

Hawkley, L.C. & Cacioppo, J.T. (2010). Loneliness matters: A theoretical and empirical review of consequences and mechanisms. *Annals of Behavioral Medicine*, 40(2), 219. https://doi.org/10.1007/s12160-010-9210-8.

Hole, J., Hirsch, M., Ball, E. & Meads, C. (2015). Music as an aid for postoperative recovery in adults: A systematic review and meta-analysis. *The Lancet*, 386(10004), 659–1671. doi: https://doi.org/10.1016/S0140-6736(15)60169-6.

Institute for Music and Neurologic Function (2007). *Rhythmic Activities for Everyday Care, a Dementia Care Video Training Guide*. New York, NY: IMNF.

International Association for Music and Medicine (2020). *Music Therapy in the Context of Dementia: People with Dementia and their Caregivers*, Webinar, IAMM, July 22, 2020.

Kolanowski, A., Fick, D., Frazer, C, & Penrod, J. (2010). It's about time: Use of nonpharmacological interventions in the nursing home. *Journal of Nursing Scholarship*, 42(2), 214–222. doi:10.1111/j.1547-5069.2010.01338.x

Koenig, J. (2021). *The Musical Child: Using the Power of Music to Raise Children who are Happy, Healthy, and Whole*. Boston, MA: Houghton Mifflin.

KPMG (2021). Alzheimer's Disease and Music Engagement Economic Impact Analysis, NeuroArts Blueprint Initiative, 2021, available at https://neuroartsblueprint.org.

Kraus, N. (2021). *Of Sound Mind: How Our Brain Constructs a Meaningful Sonic World*. Cambridge, MA: The MIT Press.

Kroenke, K., Strine, T.W., Spritzer, R.L., Williams, J.B., Berry, J.T. & Mokdad, A.H. (2009). The PHQ-8 as a measure of current depression in the general population. *Journal of Affective Disorders*, 114(1–3), 163–173.

Ladányi, E., Persici, V., Fiveash, A., Tillmann, B. & Gordon, R.L. (2020). Is atypical rhythm a risk factor for developmental speech and language disorders? *Wiley Interdisciplinary Reviews: Cognitive Science*, 11(5):e1528. doi: 10.1002/wcs.1528.

Lin, Yu *et al.* (2011). Effectiveness of group music intervention against agitated behavior in elderly persons with dementia. *International Journal of Geriatric Psychiatry*, 26(7), 670–678.

Loewy, J. (2020). Music therapy as a potential intervention for sleep improvement. *Nature and Science of Sleep*, 12, 1–9. https://doi.org/10.2147/NSS.S194938.

Luria, A.R. (1971 Russian edition; 1987). *The Man with a Shattered World*. Cambridge, MA: Harvard University Press.

MacDonald, R.A.R. (2013). Music, health, and well-being: A review. *International Journal of Qualitative Studies on Health and Well-being*, 8(1), 20635. doi: 10.3402/qhw.v8io.20635.

Magee, W.L. (2013). Models for Roles and Collaborations when Using Music Technology in Music Therapy. In W.L. Magee (ed.), *Music Technology in Therapeutic and Health Settings* (p.363). London: Jessica Kingsley Publishers.

Mas-Herrero, E., Singer, N., Ferreri, L., McPhee, M., Zatorre, R. & Ripollés, P. (2020). Rock 'n' roll but not sex or drugs: Music is negatively correlated to depressive symptoms during the COVID-19 pandemic via reward-related mechanisms. https://psyarxiv.com/x5upn.

Meadows, G. & McLennan, H. (2022). *Power of Music*. Report of UK Music and Music for Dementia. London: UK Music.

Mittleman, M.S. & Papayannopoulou, P.M. (2018). Editorial: The Unforgettables: A chorus for people with dementia with their family members and friends. *International Psychogeriatrics*, 30(6), 779–789. doi: 10.1017/S1041610217001867.

Murthy, V.H. (2020). *Together: The Healing Power of Human Connection in a Sometimes Lonely World*. New York, NY: HarperCollins Publishers.

Nagler, J. (1998). Digital Music Technology in Music Therapy Practice. In C.M. Tomaino, *Clinical Applications of Music Therapy in Neurologic Rehabilitation*. St Louis, Missouri: MMB Music Publisher.

National Academies of Sciences, Engineering, and Medicine (2020). *Social Isolation and Loneliness in Older Adults: Opportunities for the Health Care System.* Washington, DC: The National Academies Press.

National Organization for Arts in Health. (2017, September). *Arts, Health, & Wellbeing in America.* Retrieved August 16, 2021, from https://thenoah.net/wp-content/uploads/2019/01/NOAH-2017-White-Paper-Online-Edition.pdf, Cited in *NeuroArts Blueprint: Advancing the Science of Arts, Health, and Wellbeing*, The Aspen Institute, 2021, p. 83.

National Institute on Aging of the NIH (2019). Participating in the arts creates paths to healthy aging. www.nia.nih.gov/news/participating-arts-creates-paths-healthy-aging, accessed on 3 October, 2023.

Norton, A., Zipse, L., Marchina, S. & Schlaug, G. (2009). Melodic intonation therapy: Shared insights on how it is done and why it might help. *Annals of the New York Academy of Sciences*, 1169, 431–436.

Paul, S. & Ramsey, D. (2000). Music therapy in physical medicine and rehabilitation. *Australian Occupational Therapy Journal*, 47(3), 111–118. https://doi.org/10.1046/j.1440-1630.2000.00215.x.

Powell, T. (2019). *Dementia Reimagined: Building a Life of Joy and Dignity from Beginning to End.* New York, NY: Avery, an imprint of Penguin Random House LLC.

Ramsey, D. (2002). The restoration of communal experiences during the group music therapy process with non-fluent aphasic patients. Submitted in partial fulfillment of the requirement for the Doctor of Arts, School of Education, New York University.

Reynolds, G. (2021). How exercise assists aging brains. *The New York Times*, March 3, 2021.

Rogers, A. & Fleming, P. (1981). Rhythm and melody in speech therapy for the neurologically impaired. *Music Therapy*, 1(1), 33–38.

Sacks, O. (1985). *The Man Who Mistook his Wife for a Hat.* London: Picador.

Sacks, O. (1990). *Awakenings.* New York, NY: HarperPerennial.

Sacks, O. (1991). Statement at Forever Young: Music and Aging, Hearing before the Special Committee on Aging, United States Senate, 102nd Congress, First Session; Washington, DC, August 1, 1991.

Sacks, O. (2007). *Musicophilia: Tales of Music and the Brain.* New York, NY: Alfred A. Knopf.

Sample, I. (2016). Breakthrough in understanding chills and thrills of musical rapture. *The Guardian.* www.theguardian.com/science/2016/jun/17/breakghrough-in-understanding-the-chills-and-thrills of-musical-rapture, accessed on December 10, 2021.

Schlaug, G., Norton, A., Ozdemir, E. & Helm-Estabrook, N. (2007). Long-term neural and behavioral effects of melodic intonation therapy in patients with chronic Broca's aphasia. *Neurology*, 68(1), A177.

Sengupta, M., Lendon, J.P., Caffrey, C., Melekin, A. & Singh, P. (2022). Post-acute and long-term care providers and services users in the United States, 2017–2018. National Center for Health Statistics. *Vital Health Stat*, 3(47). doi: https://dx.doi.org/10.15620/cdc:115346.

Solomon, A. (2015, paperback). *The Noonday Demon: An Atlas of Depression.* New York, NY: Scriber Books.

Stoewen, D.L. (2015). Health and wellness. *The Canadian Veterinary Journal*, 56(9), 983–984.

Taladrid, S. (2020). Meet the Italians making music together under coronavirus quarantine. *The New Yorker*, Video Department, March 19, 2020.

Thaut, M.H. (2005). *Rhythm, Music, and the Brain: Scientific Foundations and Clinical Applications*. New York, NY: Routledge.

Tomaino, C. (2002). How music can reach the silenced brain. *Cerebrum*, 4(1), 22–33, published by The Dana Forum on Brain Science.

Tomaino, C., Kim, M., Butler, L. & Sobol, M. (2008). *Therapeutic Drumming and Rhythmic Activities for Nursing Home Residents with Dementia: A Dissemination Project*. Training booklet and video. New York State Department of Health, Electronic Dementia Guide for Excellence (EDGE) Project.

Tomaino, C. & Wilkens, J. (1996). The role of melody and rhythm in the rehabilitation of persons with dysarthria. Unpublished report to the Haym Salomon Foundation.

Truschel, J. (2022). Depression Definition and DSM-5 Diagnostic Criteria. Psychom. www.psycom.net/depression/major-depressive-disorder/dsm-5-depression-criteria, accessed on February 26, 2023.

Vaillant, G.E. (1977). *Adaptation to Life*. Boston, MA: Little, Brown and Company.

Verghase, J. et al. (2003). Leisure activities and the risk of dementia in the elderly. *New England Journal of Medicine*, 348, 2508–2516. doi: 10.1056/NEJMoa022252.

Villarroel, M.A. & Terlizzi, E.P. (2020). Symptoms of depression among adults: United States, 2019. NCHS Data Brief, no 379. Hyattsville, MD: National Center for Health Statistics.

WHO (1948)Preamble to the Constitution of the World Health Organization as adopted by the International Health Conference, New York, 19-22 June, 1946, signed on 22 July 1946 by representatives of 61 States (Official Records of the World Health Organization, no. 2, p.100) and entered into force on 7 April 1948.

WHO (2022) Key Facts, June 17. www.who.int/news-room/fact-sheets/detail/mental-health-strengthening-our-response, accessed on July 25, 2023.

Wolf, L. & Wolf, T. (2011). Music and health care: A paper commissioned by the Musical Connections Program of Carnegie Hall's Weill Music Institute.